Contents

List of tables, figures and boxes

Tables

Figures

Boxes

REVISED SECOND EDITION

THE HEALTH AND SOCIAL CARE DIVIDE

The experiences of older people

Jon Gl

Consul

The POL

PfL

PRESS

In memory of Marjorie Fielding (1916-1996)
and for Les and Gladys.

First published in Great Britain in May 2004 by

The Policy Press
University of Bristol
Fourth Floor
Beacon House
Queen's Road
Bristol BS8 1QU
UK

Tel +44 (0)117 331 4054
Fax +44 (0)117 331 4093
e-mail tpp-info@bristol.ac.uk
www.policypress.org.uk

British Library Cataloguing in Publication Data
A catalogue record for this book is available from the British Library.

Library of Congress Cataloging-in-Publication Data
A catalog record for this book has been requested.

ISBN 1 86134 525 9 paperback

Reprinted 2005

A hardcover version of this book is also available

Jon Glasby is a qualified social worker and Senior Lecturer in the Health Services
Management Centre, and **Rosemary Littlechild** is a Lecturer in Social Work in the
Institute of Applied Social Studies, both at the University of Birmingham.

The right of **Jon Glasby** and **Rosemary Littlechild** to be identified as authors of
this work has been asserted by them in accordance with the 1988 Copyright,
Designs and Patents Act.

Cover design by Qube Design Associates, Bristol.
Front cover: photograph supplied by kind permission of www.JohnBirdsall.co.uk
Printed and bound in Great Britain by Hobbs the Printers Ltd, Southampton.

Preface

This book is intended to provide a human face to some of the many research findings that point towards the problematic nature of the health and social care divide. The case studies included here are composites compiled from the experiences of people whose lives have been severely affected, often for the worse, by the issues discussed. This book is testimony to their suffering, courage and endurance.

Acknowledgements

Thanks to our colleagues at the University of Birmingham for their comments and suggestions, and to practitioners in a range of health and social care settings for their input, advice and experience. We are particularly grateful to The Policy Press for all their help and support and to PEPAR Publications (the publishers of the first edition of this book).

We are also grateful to Professor Caroline Glendinning and Professor Jill Manthorpe for their comments and support with early proposals and drafts.

ONE

Introduction

Since coming to power in May 1997, the New Labour government has pledged its commitment to bringing down 'the Berlin Wall' that has developed between health and social services (DoH, 1998a). This may seem like dramatic language, but the problematic nature of the division between these two public agencies has been one of the most controversial and enduring issues of modern British social policy. For frontline workers, the need to overcome a tangle of legal, administrative and organisational obstacles in order to work effectively across service boundaries with colleagues from other professions and backgrounds is an almost daily struggle. Be it hospital discharge, continuing care, domiciliary care or rehabilitation, the boundaries between these services are an almost constant source of difficulty, debate and consternation. For individual service users who find themselves trapped between these two large and powerful agencies, the experience is frequently one of frustration, disillusionment and despair. In extreme cases, it is not unknown for a patient to fail to meet the criteria for either health or social care, falling between the boundaries of existing service provision and being passed backwards and forwards until a major crisis occurs. The dangers of this have recently been recognised by the government, which has pledged its commitment to supporting more effective joint working between health and social services. As part of this process, a wide range of new policy initiatives has been introduced, many of which will significantly affect the work of frontline practitioners, but have not yet become widely known at ground level.

Against this background, this book seeks to provide an easily comprehensible introduction to policy and practice at the interface between health and social care. Chapter Two begins with an introduction to partnership working between health and social services, exploring the rationale for working together and some of the factors that help and hinder. Next, Chapter Three explores the legal and policy context, providing a chronological overview of developments in the field of health and social care provision since the Second World War. Chapters Four to Nine examine key issues from practice, combining a review of the existing research with detailed case studies compiled from a number of examples from practice. These case studies are designed to provide a human face to the various administrative and professional difficulties that are often involved in multidisciplinary working. Although the health and social care divide is a difficult issue for the workers involved, they should never lose sight of the human suffering that can be caused by the failure of service providers to collaborate effectively. Aimed at students, frontline workers and first-line managers, each chapter concludes with good practice guidelines and guidance on further reading for those interested in following up particular issues in more detail. Throughout, the book contains a number of reflective exercises so that readers can take time out from the text and consider how the issues raised can be translated and applied to their own situations and work places. Finally, the book concludes by summarising key implications for policy and practice and provides details of how to access relevant websites.

Although many of the issues highlighted here are applicable to a range of community care user groups, analysis focuses specifically on the experiences of older people. This is the result of six main factors:

- Older people are major consumers of health and social services, with estimates of the amount of money spent on community care services for this user group ranging from 47-82% of total public expenditure on health and social services (Victor, 1997, pp 91-2).
- Older people often have multiple and complex health needs, straddling the boundaries of traditional service provision (Sidell, 1995).
- Demographic changes mean that the number of older people has increased dramatically and is set to carry on rising. Since the turn of the 20th century, the number of older people has risen by 400% and is forecast to continue to grow until at least 2030. By far the most significant increase will be in the number of people aged 85+, who will be three times more numerous in 2050 than in the 1990s (Royal Commission on Long Term Care, 1999). These changes will clearly impact upon health and social services, placing greater strain on the current system and forcing practitioners to consider new ways of working.
- Older people have been slower than other client groups to form a user group or movement to represent their interests. Attempts to involve older people in service planning or delivery have also been few and far between (Barnes, 1998).
- Some older people are particularly prone to poverty and poor housing (Tinker, 1997), and lack the resources to aid recovery from illness or to make alternative provision for their needs.
- Work with older people has traditionally been seen as a low priority (Bowl, 1986; Marshall, 1990; Means and Smith, 1998a), attracting fewer recruits and being perceived as 'unglamorous' work suitable only for less qualified workers.

For all these reasons, older service users are particularly vulnerable when divisions emerge between health and social service providers. Despite this, many of the issues discussed and the policy initiatives reviewed will also be of relevance to other user groups. Thus, while partnership working initiatives often focus on older people, we know that people with mental health problems (Hancock et al, 1997; Glasby et al, 2003), people with learning difficulties (DoH, 2002a; Towell, 2002), people with physical impairments (Glasby and Littlechild, 2002; RADAR, 2003) and children and young people (Watson et al, 2002; DfES/DoH, 2003; HM Treasury, 2003; Laming, 2003) all have needs which require a multi-agency response. Similarly, the partnership working themes and issues explored later in Chapter Two within the context of health and social care may also be applicable to other areas of social policy such as housing, regeneration, public health, crime and disorder, substance misuse and promoting social inclusion (see, for example, Balloch and Taylor, 2001; Glendinning et al, 2002a).

Throughout this book, we focus on partnership working or interagency collaboration between health and social care as a means to an end (that is, as a means to better services, experiences and outcomes for service users and carers). In the current policy context, we feel that there is a danger that partnerships are seen as an automatic policy response to all kinds of issues and problems – almost to the extent that they become an end in themselves. While we welcome the current emphasis on services working more effectively together, we feel that partnerships should be the means by which we improve things for individual service users like the ones whose cases are cited in Chapters Four to Nine of this book – if partnerships do not lead to improvements for users and carers, then they are part of the problem rather than part of the solution. Although we acknowledge that frontline health and social care agencies are often doing their best to work together in difficult circumstances, we support a summary of the current situation provided by a Department of Health discussion document, *Partnership in action* (DoH, 1998a, p 3):

> All too often when people have complex needs spanning both health and social care good quality services are sacrificed for sterile arguments about boundaries. When this happens people, often the most vulnerable in our society ... and those who care for them find themselves in the no man's land between health and social services. This is not what people want or need. It places the needs of the organisation above the needs of the people they are there to serve. It is poor organisation, poor practice, poor use of taxpayers' money – it is unacceptable.

It is what this poor practice means for service users and their carers and what workers can do to improve the situation that is the focus of the remainder of this book.

TWO

Partnership working in health and social care

By way of introduction, this chapter explores some of the wider literature on relationships between health and social care and on partnership working to consider issues such as:

- the meaning of partnership working;
- the reasons for working in partnership;
- the prevalence of partnerships;
- factors that help and hinder partnerships.

What is partnership working?

Exercise A: Partnership working

1. Think of as many different terms as you can for 'partnership working' (multidisciplinary working or interagency collaboration are two examples).
2. Is it possible to distinguish what each of these terms means or how they differ from each other, or are they used interchangeably?

   As an example, Lacey (2001, pp 8-13) describes how some commentators distinguish between *multidisciplinary* (professionals from more than one discipline working alongside but separately from each other), *interdisciplinary* (professionals sharing information and making decisions about support services, but working separately and implementing care independently of each other) and *trans-disciplinary* working (the sharing of information and skills across professional boundaries to allow one or two team members to be the primary workers supported by others working as consultants).

3. However, how meaningful are these distinctions from the point of view of students, frontline workers or services users?

Partnership working between health and social care is a central feature of current government policy and the focus of a significant range of activities at a local level. Although there has long been a recognition of the need for interagency collaboration to provide seamless services for users and carers (see, for example, Means and Smith, 1998b; Lewis, 2001; see also Chapter Three of this book), this has acquired increasing impetus following the commitment of the New Labour government to achieving 'joined-up solutions' to 'joined-up problems'.

Responding to this central agenda, a large number of different partnership arrangements are being developed in different parts of the country, spawning a series of new ways of working and new types of health and social care organisations (see Chapter Three of this book for further details).

Although there is a substantial and growing literature on partnership working, most of the available texts are beset by difficulties of terminology and of definition. Not only are there a large number of different terms in use, but also different writers tend to employ them in different ways (see Exercise A). As an example, Leathard (1994, p 5) lists 52 different definitions, describing this area as "a terminological quagmire".

For Sullivan and Skelcher (2002), partnership working can be defined by its emphasis on:

- a shared responsibility for assessing the need for action, determining the type of action to be taken and agreeing the means of implementation;
- negotiation between people from different agencies committed to working together over more than the short term;
- an intention to secure the delivery of benefits or added value which could not have been provided by a single agency acting alone.

For the government spending watchdog, the Audit Commission (2002a, p 10),

- services should be organised around the user;
- all of the players should recognise that they are interdependent and understand that action in one part of the system has an impact elsewhere;
- the following are all shared: vision; objectives; action, including redesigning services; resources; risk;
- users experience services as seamless and the boundaries between organisations are not apparent to them.

Further definitions are set out in Box 2.1.

Box 2.1: Defining partnerships

A minimal definition [of partnership working] would require the involvement of at least two agents or agencies with at least some common interests or interdependencies; and would also probably require a relationship between them that involves a degree of trust, equality or reciprocity.... Implicit in this definition ... is the requirement that partnerships are characterised by a degree of autonomy on the part of relatively equal partners to determine and implement a plan or programme. (Glendinning et al, 2002a, p 3)

The 'integration' of health, social care, and related services (for example, housing and transportation), particularly for vulnerable groups such as the frail elderly, has become a recurring theme in the development of health and social care policy in the UK. The term 'integrated care' has been given many definitions ..., most of which concentrate on the design and development of techniques and models to establish both informal and formal collaboration between the health and social care sectors. Such integration can occur at many different levels, including planning and policy making, funding, administration, and the provision and delivery of care itself. (Goodwin and Shapiro, 2001, p 1)

Interprofessional working is ... defined as 'how two or more people from different professions communicate and cooperate to achieve a common goal'. (Øvretveit et al, 1997, p 2)

[Partnership working is] the search to connect the health care system (acute, primary, medical and skilled) with other human service systems (eg long-term care, education, and vocational and housing services) in order to improve outcomes (clinical, satisfaction, and efficiency). (Leutz, 1999, p 78)

Indeed, such is the confusing array of terms available that some commentators have questioned how useful or meaningful concepts such as 'partnership working' may be. As Banks (2002, p 5) explains:

> The term 'partnerships' is increasingly losing credibility, as it has become a catch-all for a wide range of concepts and a panacea for a multitude of ills. Partnerships can cover a wide spectrum of relationships and can operate at different levels, from informally taking account of other players, to having a constructive dialogue, working together on a project or service, joint commissioning and strategic alliances.

Despite this, the vast majority of commentators continue to employ terms such as 'joint working', 'partnership' and 'interagency collaboration', using these phrases as a sort of shorthand to describe a way of working which is characterised by:

- a desire to achieve benefits that could not be attained by a single agency working by itself;
- a recognition that some services are interdependent and that action in one part of the system will have a 'knock-on effect' somewhere else;
- some sort of shared vision of the way forward or shared purpose.

For us, the issue is not so much one of definition; rather, it is how to create an appropriate level of 'joint-ness' or coherence within health and social services so that users and carers experience them as a consistent and coordinated package rather than as fragmented and disjointed. Of course, achieving this 'joint-ness' depends on action at a number of different levels and can require a number of different types of joint working. For example, Poxton (2003) suggests that health and social care are increasingly being required to work together at three different levels:

1. At a *strategic level*, agencies are required to plan together and share information about the use of resources, for example through Health Improvement and Modernisation Plans and Joint Investment Plans (see Chapter Three of this book).
2. At the level of *operational management*, a range of policies require a demonstration of partnership. For example, the *National service framework for older people* requires the implementation of a single assessment process that covers health and social care needs (see Chapter Three).
3. At the level of *individual care and support*, these operational requirements are taken further with expectations of a single point of access, shared information systems and joint training across health and social care staff.

In addition, Poxton (2003) identifies a spectrum of partnership working, which can include a wide range of different activities and approaches, depending on the nature of the partnership concerned and the outcome being sought:

*   *communication* – informing each other of separate actions;
*   *coordination* – working separately but mindful of each other's actions;
*   *collaboration* – working together in a cohesive way;
*   *integration* – working together as one agency.

A similar model is suggested by Pratt et al (1998), who distinguish between different types of relationship based on *competition* (desiring to improve individual performance), *cooperation* (working with others, even if sometimes out of self-interest), *collaboration* (working together towards a shared goal) and *co-evolution* (where partners are committed to co-designing something together for a shared purpose).

Why work in partnership?

In the same way that the partnership literature contains a myriad of different terms and definitions, so, too, many commentators cite a wide range of different reasons why health and social care agencies (and other organisations as well) should be seeking to work together. According to one account (Audit Commission, 1998), for example, partnership working can help to:

*   deliver coordinated packages of services to individuals;
*   tackle so-called 'wicked issues';[1]
*   reduce the impact of organisational fragmentation;

Exercise B: Why work in partnership?

1. Drawing on your existing knowledge of health and social care services, identify examples of partnership projects or approaches and think about the reasons behind these partnerships – what are they trying to achieve?

2. What impact could a partnership approach between health and social care have for:

- children and young people?
- people with physical impairments?
- people with mental health problems?
- older people?
- people with learning difficulties?

- people living in poverty?
- people with HIV/AIDS?
- homeless people?
- family carers?

For example, one local authority is working with NHS partners to develop a new, integrated team made up of housing, welfare rights, leisure, social care and NHS workers to meet the needs of local older people. The aim is to provide a single point of access, to reduce duplication and to provide more appropriate responses to the needs of service users. As a result, it is anticipated that the team will be able to respond to requests for assistance more quickly than in the past and in a more holistic manner, thereby intervening at an early stage and preventing future crises from occurring in older people's health.

- bid for, or gain access to, new resources;
- meet a statutory requirement (see Chapter Three of this book for further details of statutory requirements);
- align services provided by all partners with the needs of users;
- make better use of resources;
- stimulate more creative approaches to problems;
- influence the behaviour of the partners or of third parties in ways that none of the partners acting alone could achieve.

At a team level, moreover, Payne (2000, p 41) highlights the importance of multi-professional working as a means of bringing together skills, sharing information, achieving greater continuity of care, apportioning and ensuring responsibility and accountability, and coordinating resources. At a more colloquial level, this can perhaps be encapsulated by the concept of the 'whole as being greater than the sum of its parts'.

A useful distinction is also made by Goodwin and Shapiro (2001, p 1), who suggest that the rationale for partnership working can be divided into those factors that are based on *organisational objectives* (the advantages of integrating health and social care organisations and systems) and *service objectives* (the advantages of integrating care provision to service users and patients) (Box 2.2).

Box 2.2: The rationale for partnership working

Organisational objectives:
- Reducing duplication.
- Streamlining management functions and maximising value for money.
- Streamlining accountability.
- Integrating budgets.
- Integrating to overcome organisational and cultural barriers to partnership.
- Developing a common vision and a shared plan.
- Engaging users and carers.

Service objectives:
- Changing existing service patterns to meet need more appropriately.
- Identifying gaps in provision and addressing unmet need.
- Promoting easier access for users and carers through a 'seamless' service.
- Engendering a common approach to the provision of services.
- Improving the patient/carer experience of the care process. (Goodwin and Shapiro, 2001, p 1)

While it is not within the remit of this book to examine these claims in more detail, it is important to sound a note of caution. Although the rationales for partnership working cited above seem very plausible, the evidence base on which such statements are made is not always as sound as it could be. Often, much of the partnership working literature is very 'faith based' – asserting that partnership working is a 'good thing' without necessarily citing any evidence to support such claims. While partnership working certainly seems like a commonsense idea (and certainly can bring a range of benefits), it is important to retain a critical approach to the literature and to ask on an ongoing basis questions such as:

- What is my agency (and others) trying to achieve?
- What is the best way of achieving this goal?

On many occasions, the answer to the second question may involve a conscious decision that some form of partnership is the best way to proceed. If so, agencies will have a clearly articulated goal that they wish to achieve and a proposed method of meeting this desired end (and hence a working hypothesis about the best way forward that they can test out in practice – that is, did the partnership achieve what we wanted it to?). This is effectively a form of evaluation that will allow frontline workers and the organisations they work for to engage in partnerships that meet their stated aims and, as we suggested in the introduction to this book, ensure that all partnerships are means to an end rather than ends in themselves.

In many ways, this book represents a stage before the process outlined earlier. In Chapters Four to Nine, we cite a number of real-life case studies that illustrate the problems that can arise when services do not work together and the benefits that can result when they do, setting out some good practice guidance based on the experience of the individual older people concerned. Thus, the evidence that emerges with regard to the need for partnership working is based not on government policy documents or faith-based literature, but on the personal testimony and experiences of real people in real-life situations.

The prevalence of partnerships

Exercise C: The prevalence of partnerships

For existing practitioners and managers:
1. Drawing on your current knowledge of health and social care services, list all the partnerships that exist in the area where you live/work.
2. How many people work in these partnership projects?
3. How many service users and carers do these projects serve?
4. How much money is invested in health and social care partnerships?
5. How much management time is devoted to improving local partnerships?

For students and other readers:
1. Read a recent issue of a weekly health or social care publication (examples might include *Community Care* or the *Health Service Journal*).
2. How many of the articles and/or job adverts refer to partnership initiatives?
3. What impression does this give you about the scope and scale of partnership working?

As a result of many of the factors highlighted earlier, there has been a substantial increase in the number and scope of partnerships in recent years. According to a Local Government Association (2000) survey sent to all 410 local authorities in England and Wales, for example, over four out of five respondents rated their relationship with the health service as positive, with over nine out of ten suggesting that this relationship had improved over the last three years. A total of 71% of local authorities reported existing partnership arrangements with health services (although this figure rose to 98% when focusing only on unitary and shire counties – authorities which provide social care services).

In addition, research conducted by Sullivan and Skelcher (2002) suggests that there are around 5,500 individual partnership bodies at a local or regional level stimulated or directly created by government in England, Scotland, Wales and Northern Ireland. These can be divided into around 60 types of different partnerships from health improvement to regeneration, and from child development to rural transport. Partnerships may spend around £15-20 billion per year, with up to 75,000 places on partnership boards (compared to 23,000 local councillors and 60,000 members of quangos). Large though these figures may sound, Sullivan and Skelcher are at pains to emphasise that such numbers may well be an underestimate of the true extent of partnership working.

Whatever the true number of partnerships, the key point is that partnership working is a vast and rapidly expanding arena, commanding significant resources and occupying significant management time. Indeed, sometimes there may even be concerns that there are too many partnerships – diluting and fragmenting practitioners' and managers' time across too many areas and priorities. Whatever your point of view, however, the overall issue is clear: there is a growing recognition of the need for different agencies to come together in a whole host of new ways, and this is likely to have significant implications for frontline practitioners.

Factors that help and hinder partnerships

Exercise D: Factors that help and hinder partnerships

1. Think of a situation where you have worked with someone from a different agency or professional background to yourself. If you are a practitioner or manager, try to concentrate on an example involving a health and social partnership. If you are a student, choose any situation where you have to work with another person to achieve a particular task (for example, working in a group at school or at university, being in a sports team, and so on).
2. Where this relationship or encounter worked well, what were the underlying factors that helped the situation to work?
3. Where this relationship or encounter worked badly, what were the underlying barriers that got in the way?

Just as the partnership literature has many different definitions of partnership working and rationales for working together, it also offers considerable advice as to the factors that help and hinder partnership working. Since the early 1990s, a key contributor has been the Nuffield Institute for Health at the University of Leeds, whose research is cited frequently throughout the remainder of this book. Throughout a series of studies, researchers there have identified a number of barriers to interagency collaboration and principles for more effective partnerships (Box 2.3). Many of these are echoed by Poxton (2003), whose Partnership Readiness Framework seeks to identify those factors that need to be in place and/or considered by local agencies that wish to develop effective partnerships (Box 2.4).

For the Audit Commission (2002a), partnership working is aided by investing time to build good relationships; developing a strategic vision of the way forward; mapping current services and redesigning where appropriate; leadership; an open and flexible organisational culture; shared information; a single assessment of

Box 2.3: Partnership working: what helps and what hinders?

Barriers:
- *Structural* (the fragmentation of service responsibilities across and within agency boundaries).
- *Procedural* (differences in planning and budget cycles).
- *Financial* (differences in funding mechanisms and resource flows).
- *Professional* (differences in ideologies, values and professional interests).
- *Perceived threats to status, autonomy and legitimacy.*

Principles for strengthening strategic approaches to collaboration:
- *Shared vision:* specifying what is to be achieved in terms of user-centred goals, clarifying the purpose of collaboration as a mechanism for achieving such goals, and mobilising commitment around goals, outcomes and mechanisms.
- *Clarity of roles and responsibilities:* specifying and agreeing 'who does what', and designing organisational arrangements by which roles and responsibilities are to be fulfilled.
- *Appropriate incentives and rewards:* promoting organisational behaviour consistent with agreed goals and responsibilities, and harnessing organisational self-interest to collective goals.
- *Accountability for joint working:* monitoring achievements in relation to the stated vision, holding individuals and agencies to account for the fulfilment of pre-determined roles and responsibilities, and providing feedback and review of vision, responsibilities, incentives, and their inter-relationship. (Hudson et al, 1997)

Box 2.4: The Partnership Readiness Framework

- Building shared values and principles.
- Agreeing specific policy shifts.
- Being prepared to explore new service options.
- Determining agreed boundaries.
- Agreeing respective roles with regard to commissioning, purchasing and providing.
- Identifying agreed resource pools.
- Ensuring effective leadership.
- Providing sufficient development capacity.
- Developing and sustaining good personal relationships.
- Paying specific attention to mutual trust and attitude. (Poxton, 2003)

needs; a joined-up approach to workforce development; and the creation of multi-professional teams. In addition, a further list of barriers and success factors is provided in a national survey conducted by the Local Government Association (2000). These include:

Success factors

- The current emphasis on partnership working in policy documents.
- A sense of shared/complementary roles, aims and priorities.
- Good working relations between key personnel.
- Local authority representation in Primary Care Groups (PCGs) (now Primary Care Trusts or PCTs) (see Chapter Three of this book).
- Senior commitment to partnership working.
- The presence of key 'champions' or 'personalities'.
- A history of joint working.
- Additional funding made available for particular partnership initiatives.
- Shared boundaries.
- Political support from council members.

Barriers

- Budgetary problems and financial differences between health and social care.
- Lack of understanding of each other's roles, cultures, processes and language.
- Differences in the medical and social models of care.
- The disruption caused by large-scale reorganisations.
- Rapid staff turnover and poor interpersonal relationships (characterised by suspicious or competitive behaviour).
- A lack of time and human resources.
- A lack of common geographical boundaries.
- National priorities for the NHS versus local priorities for local government.

Interestingly, fewer than 10 authorities (out of a total of 297 responding to the survey) reported a lack of willingness on either side to work in partnership. Overall, however, participants in the survey were keen to emphasise that these success factors and barriers by themselves were not enough to help/hinder effective partnerships: ultimately, what was needed was considerable effort and commitment from partner agencies. As one local authority observed (quoted in Local Government Association, 2000, pp 18-19):

> To achieve [good partnership working] requires good relationships and trust between the agencies responsible for frontline services, so that sensible multidisciplinary cooperation results: social workers, nurses, therapists, home carers and GPs working together in flexible

ways according to an individual's needs. Developing such arrangements takes a considerable investment of time and money.... The scale of the task in management, culture and organisational terms should not be underestimated.

Finally, Glasby's (2003a) research into delayed hospital discharges (Figure 2.1; see also Chapter Four of this book) identifies three different levels of activity which health and social care agencies need to address in order to develop effective partnerships: individual (I), organisational (O) and structural (S). While there is much more that can be done to encourage joint working between individual practitioners and local health and social care organisations (the I and O levels), Glasby argues that more action is required at a central government level to tackle some of the legal, administrative and bureaucratic barriers to partnership working. These are deeply engrained in our current service structures and, ultimately, derive from the fact that the current health and social care system is based on an underlying division between two very different organisations with different priorities, values and ways of working. The framework is presented in terms of a series of interlocking circles, as each level of activity has the capacity to influence or be reinforced by the others. Thus, the way in which individuals behave is based in part on the norms, values and policies of their organisations, which in turn are shaped by a series of structural barriers to partnership working at a central government level. Similarly, these structural barriers depend in part on the characteristics of particular types of health and social care organisation, which depend ultimately on the people working in these organisations. As a result, any policy designed to achieve true partnership working will need to operate at all three levels of activity at the same time if it is to be successful.

Figure 2.1: Different levels of partnership working

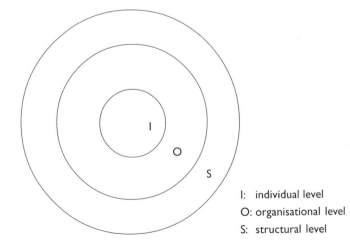

I: individual level
O: organisational level
S: structural level

Source: Glasby (2003a)

Summary

Partnership working between health and social care is a key government priority and is rapidly becoming a key feature of local health and social care delivery. Unfortunately, much of the existing partnership working literature is often very faith based and the underlying assumption that partnership is 'a good thing' (while quite possibly true) needs further investigation and research. In spite of this, there is nevertheless a large and growing body of knowledge and literature that attempts to explore the concept of health and social care partnerships. Although there are a large number of different approaches to the topic, key features of many current definitions of partnership include:

- a desire to achieve benefits which could not be attained by a single agency working by itself;
- a recognition that some services are interdependent and that action in one part of the system will have a 'knock-on effect' somewhere else;
- some sort of shared vision of the way forward or shared purpose.

In seeking to promote more effective partnerships, moreover, much of the literature emphasises the importance of factors such as trust, shared vision and good interpersonal relationships in order to overcome the financial, professional, structural and procedural barriers to interagency collaboration. Above all, however, there is a growing recognition that partnership working is no longer an option but a requirement. Health and social care services need to work together to a much greater extent than in the past if service users and carers are to receive coordinated and coherent packages of care which meet the diversity and totality of their needs. People do not live their lives according to the categories we create in our public services, and this is something that requires a response from health and social care practitioners and organisations. It is the nature and impact of this response that is the focus of the rest of this book, both in terms of official policy (Chapter Three) and individual practice (Chapters Four to Nine).

Note

[1] That is, complex, crosscutting issues where we are not certain how to resolve the particular problem. Examples might include social exclusion or substance misuse.

Further reading

In recognition of the increasing importance of partnership working, a growing number of introductory textbooks are beginning to appear which offer useful overviews of many of the issues at stake. Key sources include:

- 6, P., Leat, D., Seltzer, K. and Stoker, G. (2002) *Towards holistic governance: The new reform agenda*, Basingstoke: Palgrave.

- Balloch, S. and Taylor, M. (eds) (2001) *Partnership working: Policy and practice*, Bristol: The Policy Press.

- Glendinning, C., Powell, M. and Rummery, K. (2002a) *Partnerships, New Labour and the governance of welfare*, Bristol: The Policy Press.

- Sullivan, H. and Skelcher, C. (2002) *Working across boundaries: Collaboration in the public services*, Basingstoke: Palgrave.

Useful information is also available from the Integrated Care Network's website (www.integratedcarenetwork.gov.uk), which explores a range of partnership topics under headings such as organisational development, policy, research, inclusion, governance and performance and evaluation.

THREE

Health and social care: the legal and policy context

Key policies summarised in this chapter include:

- National Health Service Act 1946 and National Assistance Act 1948;
- government guidance in the 1950s about residential care (circular 14/57);
- Health Service Reorganisation Act 1973;
- developments in the 1960s and 1970s such as 10-year plans, Joint Consultative Committees and joint care planning teams;
- Registered Homes Act 1984;
- *Making a reality of community care*, 1986;
- The Griffiths Report, 1988;
- *Caring for people*, 1989;
- Hospital discharge guidance, 1989;
- NHS and Community Care Act 1990;
- Community care policy and practice guidance 1990-91;
- *The patient's charter*, 1991;
- Preparing for community care, 1992-93;
- *Hospital discharge workbook*, 1994;
- Continuing care guidance, 1995;
- Funding for priority services, 1996;
- Winter pressures, 1997;
- *Better services for vulnerable people*, 1997;
- *The new NHS*, 1997;
- *Partnership in action*, 1998;
- *Modernising social services*, 1998;
- Health Act 1999;
- Royal Commission on Long Term Care, 1999;
- Ongoing developments in continuing care (the Coughlan case, 2001 guidance and the 2003 Ombudsman report);
- the government's response to the Royal Commission, 2000;
- free nursing care;
- *The NHS plan*, 2000;
- intermediate care;
- the Single Assessment Process;
- Care Trusts;
- The Health and Social Care Act 2001;
- *Shifting the balance of power*, 2001;
- The *National service framework for older people*, 2001;
- *Delivering the NHS plan*, 2002;
- hospital discharge – an ongoing issue.

In the early 21st century, attempts to encourage health and social services to work more closely together have attracted significant attention and become something of a political priority. This has resulted in a stream of policy initiatives, legislation and guidance which will inevitably affect the way practitioners work, but which have been so frequent and so numerous that many frontline workers will not yet be familiar with them. To provide an overview of recent events, this chapter offers a chronological outline of some of the key developments. While the focus is very much on changes since the introduction of the NHS and Community Care Act 1990 (NHSCCA), a brief section at the beginning touches on some of the historical antecedents of the current situation, highlighting the fact that many of today's problems and issues are by no means new. The remainder of the chapter then proceeds to examine the events associated with the passage of the NHSCCA and subsequent developments under the New Labour government elected in May 1997.

This chapter is very long, and readers may wish to use it in one of two ways according to their individual backgrounds and previous experience:

• those who want an overview of current policy and the way in which it has evolved over time may wish to read the chapter from start to finish;
• those with greater previous knowledge may wish to use this chapter as a reference guide, dipping in and out as appropriate.

Exercise E: The legal and policy context

1. Read the list of policies summarised in this chapter (see page 19).
2. Are you certain what these policy initiatives might mean for health and social care, or for your own profession/position/agency?
3. Do you know where to go to find out more about these policies?

'Early days': 1940s-1980s

In many ways, the lines of demarcation between health and social care have always been unclear, controversial and problematic. Initially, this division may well have had its origins in the now notorious Poor Law, with the sick considered blameless for their plight and hence eligible for support, and those without a recognised limiting disability being viewed as paupers undeserving of assistance (Means and Smith, 1998b). During the 19th and early 20th centuries, a rather piece-meal system emerged, with health and social care provided by a range of public, private and voluntary organisations and professionals. At this stage, there was no clear distinction between the two types of care, with local authorities providing many services which would later come to be perceived as meeting health needs (for example, community nursing, certain types of hospital and certain public health functions). While difficulties in securing collaboration between the numerous agencies involved in the provision of care services was always difficult, it was not until the Second World War that many of the divisions and issues which continue to affect service provision today began to emerge.

The 1940s

In the immediate post-war period, the **National Health Service Act 1946** and the **National Assistance Act 1948** created a system of care based on the explicit assumption that it is possible to distinguish between the *sick* (people with *health* needs who would need care from the NHS) and the *frail* (people with *social* needs who would either be cared for by their family or would enter a local authority care home). This distinction was crucial, for the former would receive their care free of charge and the latter may well be called upon to pay.

Under **Section 21** of the **National Assistance Act 1948**, all local authorities had a duty "to provide residential accommodation for persons who by reason of age, infirmity or any other circumstances are in need of care and attention which is not otherwise available to them". The key phrase here is 'care and attention', the meaning of which has caused considerable confusion and has been hotly debated ever since. Godlove and Mann (1980) have emphasised how the authors of the Act did not envisage residential homes as being equipped to provide care for people with severe mobility problems, incontinence or dementia – these were health problems that would require treatment from the NHS. However, a key feature of the development of British welfare provision since 1948 has been the extent to which residential care has been gradually redefined to include people with conditions, like those described earlier, originally conceived as health needs (Means, 1986).

The 1950s

During the 1950s, shortages of residential accommodation and the high cost of hospital care prompted a debate about the boundaries between health and social care (see also Chapter Four). In 1952, one commentator identified a 'no-man's land' between these two services, with some older people becoming stranded – "not ill enough for one, not well enough for the other" (Huws Jones, 1952, p 22). The following year, the Minister of Health (Iain Macleod) described this as "perhaps the most baffling problem in the whole of the National Health Service" (quoted in Means, 1986, p 94). Warren summarised the problem accordingly:

> There is unfortunately a wide gulf between the aids given by the Regional Hospital Board and those administered by the Local Authority. Hence the needs of the elderly frequently fall between the two bodies – the individual being not sick enough to justify

admission to a hospital and yet too disabled or frail for a vacancy in a Home. (Warren, 1951, p 106)

In response, contemporaries debated two main solutions: the creation of a half-way house between existing services or an expansion of local authority residential care to include people with greater needs. The latter option was adopted by the government and enshrined in 1957 in the **Ministry of Health Circular 14/ 57**. Henceforth, local authorities were responsible not only for 'the active older person', but also for:

- care of residents during minor illness which may require short periods in bed;
- care of the infirm (including the senile) who may require help with dressing or going to the toilet, who might be unable to manage stairs and who might need to spend part of the day in bed;
- care of terminally ill residents who would not benefit from further medical treatment.

Hospitals, however, were to remain responsible for:

- the chronic bedfast requiring nursing care over a prolonged period;
- convalescent care for older people who have completed their treatment but are not yet ready for discharge;
- confused or disturbed patients unable to live in the community or a residential home. (MoH, 1957a, 1957b).

Although this was intended to clarify responsibilities, the circular was, on its own admission, only a 'working guide' and was full of problems of interpretation:

> Could one always decide if a bedfast resident would die in three months or three years? How clear-cut was the distinction between the senile and the senile confused? At what point did spending part of the day in bed justify a resident being labelled as bedfast and thus requiring admittance to a hospital? How could one know if removal to a hospital was inhumane? (Means, 1986, p 96)

In such a situation, the circular was probably used by the different agencies involved as a bargaining device, seeking to pass as many cases as possible to the other and accepting referrals from each other only on the basis of a 'swap' (that is, a hospital would admit a sick person from residential care only if the residential home would admit a hospital patient in return) (Means and Smith, 1998b). Although later guidance sought to clarify the situation, older people were effectively placed in different types of institution not according to an assessment of their needs, but according to the balance of power between local health and social care workers (Means and Smith, 1998a, 1998b). This was to continue into the 1980s, culminating eventually in the NHSCCA. However, the bargaining process described earlier still persists to this day and the distinction between health and social care with regard to long-term care remains problematic (see later in this chapter and Chapter Six).

The 1960s and 1970s

While early debates focused on the issue of long-term care, the divide between health and social care was also significant with regard to community services (see Chapter Seven). When the National Assistance Act 1948 was passed, the focus was very much on the provision of residential care, leaving domiciliary services to voluntary organisations such as Age Concern (then the National Old People's Welfare Committee), the Red Cross and the Women's Royal Voluntary Service. Gradually, however, a division similar to the residential home versus hospital divide began to emerge, with local authority social services departments responsible for domiciliary services such as home care, meals on wheels and day care, and the NHS responsible for community health services such as health visitors and district nurses. Key events in this process included the passage of legislation such as the **Health Service Reorganisation Act 1973**, which transferred many of the community health services previously administered by local authorities to health authorities. Ongoing issues have since included the lack of coordination perceived by service users (Allen et al, 1992) and major overlaps in provision (Clarke, 1984). These issues are discussed in greater detail in Chapter Seven.

In response to some of these issues, the government devised a series of measures designed to achieve greater coordination between health and social care services. With hindsight, many of these policies have been criticised for their ineffectiveness, paving the way for some of the far-reaching reforms of the early 1990s. In particular, the amount of genuine partnership working that resulted from these initiatives is felt to have been limited by an overemphasis on structural links and processes and by the relatively small amounts of money that were involved in jointly financed projects (see, for example, Nocon, 1994; Hudson and Henwood, 2002). Key initiatives during the 1960s and 1970s included:

- In the early 1960s, **10-year plans** were introduced for hospital and community care services. These proved insufficient to promote greater coordination and were abandoned after 1966.
- In the late 1960s, the integration of the NHS into local government was briefly considered, but rejected in favour of the creation of parallel health and social care structures based on shared boundaries.
- From April 1974, the **NHS Reorganisation Act 1973** placed a statutory duty on health and local authorities to collaborate with each other through **Joint Consultative Committees**. Advisory rather than executive, these bodies

were soon seen to be inadequate for the task in hand (Wistow and Fuller, 1982), prompting calls for further reform.

- In 1976, these arrangements were strengthened by the creation of **joint care planning teams** of senior officers and by a **joint finance** programme to provide short-term funding for social services projects deemed to be beneficial to the health services. Despite growing criticisms of these mechanisms for joint working, formal arrangements for collaboration remained substantially unchanged until the community care reforms of the 1990s (Hudson et al, 1997).

The community care reforms

Despite the emphasis of the post-war services on residential, nursing and hospital provision, a reaction against institutional forms of care was to set in from the late 1950s onwards. The reasons for this were complex, but included concerns about the cost of existing services, the effectiveness of provision and the inhumane nature of some of the care provided. Of particular importance was a change in social security regulations in the early 1980s which made it easier for people with low incomes entering independent sector homes to claim **Supplementary Benefit** (now **Income Support**) towards the cost of their care. With access to this source of funding based on financial entitlement rather than any objective assessment of people's need for such a service, the number of independent residential and nursing homes rocketed:

- the number of residential and nursing home places provided by the private sector increased from 46,900 (1982) to 161,200 (1991);
- expenditure on placements in private residential/nursing homes increased from £10 million (1979) to £1,872 million (1991);
- the number of people funded by social security payments increased from 12,000 (1979) to 90,000 (1986). (Victor, 1997, p 14)

In order to regulate this area of massive growth and to restrain the social security budget, the **Registered Homes Act** was passed in 1984. This set up registration and inspection systems for residential and nursing homes, which were inspected by social services and health authorities respectively.

Against this background of growing dissatisfaction with institutional care and spiralling public expenditure, the pressure for reform began to mount, fuelled by a series of critical official reports (House of Commons Social Services Committee, 1985; Audit Commission, 1986). Ultimately, this was to culminate in a radical shake-up in the nature and focus of service provision, embodied in the passage of the NHSCCA. While these developments were the result of a complex series of factors, a key issue throughout was the failure of health and social services to provide coordinated care.

Making a reality of community care, 1986

Of all the calls for reform in the mid and late 1980s, the most significant was that of the Audit Commission. In 1986, *Making a reality of community care* provided a scathing critique of the failure of government policy to achieve care in the community. Focusing on the movement of people with mental health problems, older people and those with learning difficulties from hospital to community services, the report identified a number of underlying problems, one of which was the organisational fragmentation and confusion created by the various agencies involved in the provision of community care services. In particular, the Audit Commission drew attention to three main barriers to achieving more coordinated services:

• The confused structure of community services, with responsibility and accountability fragmented between different tiers of the NHS and within local government. Different agencies and professionals have different priorities and professional backgrounds, making greater cooperation difficult.
• Such fragmentation makes attempts to work together complex and time-consuming.
• This is exacerbated by a lack of incentives to work together and differences in organisational style.

While the report contained a number of recommendations for future policy, two in particular were of significance to the health and social care divide:

• A **single budget** should be created made up of contributions from the NHS and local authorities, but controlled by a single manager who would purchase services for older people from whichever public or private agency seemed most appropriate. The manager's activities would be overseen by a small joint board of NHS and local authority representatives. Other users, such as people with mental health problems, physical impairments or learning difficulties, should be the responsibility of a sole agency, whether it be the local authority (people with physical impairments and learning difficulties) or the NHS (people with mental health problems).
• A new, generic post of **community care worker** should be created to help with personal and social care.

Such was the seriousness of the situation that the Audit Commission called for a government review to resolve the issues it had identified.

The Griffiths Report, 1988

Heavily influenced by the Audit Commission's report, the then Secretary of State for Social Services (Norman Fowler) asked Sir Roy Griffiths to "review the way in which public funds are used to support community care policy and to advise me on the options for action that would improve the use of these funds as a contribution to a more effective community care" (Griffiths, 1988, p iii). The outcome of this review, the **Griffiths Report**, was published in March 1988 and included a series of far-reaching proposals for the reform of community care services. In essence, Griffiths proposed a new system in which social services departments would become the lead agency, assessing the community care needs of their locality, carrying out assessments of individual needs, devising packages of care to meet these needs and securing their delivery within available resources. In discharging these new duties, they should make maximum possible use of the independent sector, thereby widening consumer choice, stimulating innovation and encouraging efficiency. While these changes would inevitably impact upon the work of health and social care agencies, a number of recommendations were of particular importance for the way in which these two organisations worked together:

- Unlike the Audit Commission before him, Griffiths (1988, p 11) did not recommend the creation of a single budget to purchase community care services, rejecting "the disruption and turbulence" which major organisational and structural reform would entail. Instead, he proposed the appointment of a **Minister for Community Care** who, among other things, would draw up a definition of community care objectives and values, review progress and be seen by the public as being clearly responsible for community care.
- However, Griffiths did follow the Audit Commission in recommending the creation of **community carer** posts.
- Social services would carry out assessments and fund the care of people entering not only residential homes, but also nursing homes as well. They would also be responsible for registering and inspecting residential and non-acute nursing homes.
- Health authorities would remain responsible for medically required community health services, making any necessary input into assessing needs and delivering packages of care (Griffiths, 1988).

Although the Griffiths Report was received with a degree of cautious optimism, it was criticised on five main counts (Victor, 1997; Means and Smith, 1998a):

- it made assumptions about the ability of older people to support themselves which were not supported by research findings;
- it did not sufficiently acknowledge the burdens of caring;
- it marginalised the role of housing in community care;
- it treated the development of private sector service provision as unproblematic;
- most significantly of all, it maintained the assumption that it is possible to distinguish between health and social care, and that this division is entirely unproblematic.

Caring for people, 1989

Although the Griffiths Report was published in March 1988, the government's White Paper, *Caring for people* (DoH, 1989a) was delayed until November 1989[1]. This was thought to be because several of Griffiths' proposals sat uneasily with the government's "anti-local authority ideology" (Victor, 1997, p 17). Despite examining alternatives, the government eventually concluded that no other option was workable and the subsequent White Paper followed the majority of Griffiths' recommendations. However, major exceptions included the failure to appoint a Minister for Community Care and the rejection of the concept of a 'community carer', justified on the grounds that the role of home carers was already being expanded to include more personal care tasks (see Chapter Seven of this book). Contrary to the Griffiths Report, moreover, the registration and inspection of nursing homes was to remain the responsibility of health authorities, creating a farcical situation in which social services departments would fund nursing care, but not be able to monitor its quality.

In introducing the changes recommended by Griffiths, the government identified six key objectives:

- to promote the development of domiciliary, day and respite services;
- to ensure that service providers make support for carers a high priority;
- to make proper assessment of need the cornerstone of high quality care;
- to promote the development of a flourishing independent sector;
- to clarify the responsibilities of agencies and so make it easier to hold them to account for their performance;
- to secure better value for taxpayers' money.

To achieve the fifth aim, clarifying responsibilities, the White Paper emphasised the importance of different agencies (especially health and social services) achieving a greater degree of cooperation and coordination:

> As has been recognised in child care, it is essential that the caring services should work effectively together, each recognising and respecting the others' contribution and responsibilities. Much of this White Paper is about the clarification of those responsibilities. Nonetheless, it will continue to be essential for each of the relevant services to keep in mind the interests and responsibilities of the other; to recognise that particularly at the working interface there is much common purpose; to cross-refer cases when appropriate; and to seek and share advice and information when relevant. There is no room in community care for a narrow view of individuals' needs, nor of ways of meeting them. (DoH, 1989a, para 2.20)

In seeking to encourage effective joint working, the White Paper recognised that "Community care is about the health as well as the social needs of the population" (DoH, 1989a, para 4.1). As a result, health authorities were to remain responsible for the health needs of their locality and should set out their policies for community services, while assessments were to be multidisciplinary where appropriate and should include contributions from relevant health (and other) professionals. The government's apparent optimism that greater collaboration could be achieved appeared to be based primarily on its assertion that working closely together was mutually beneficial. To illustrate this point, it provided a number of practical examples:

> The new funding arrangements for residential care mean that discharged hospital patients will have to undergo an assessment of their care needs before the ... costs of residential accommodation can be met at public expense. Health authorities will therefore need to work with social services authorities to arrange care for elderly people who are inappropriately placed in hospital. At the same time, to make best use of their ... funds, social services authorities will need an effective primary and community health contribution to the development of domiciliary and residential care packages. (DoH, 1989a, para 6.3)

Despite this, a major criticism of the White Paper must be its continued assumption that it is possible to distinguish between health and social care needs. This was particularly the case with regard to long-term care. While the White Paper states that people requiring "continuous care for reasons of ill-health" were to remain the responsibility of health authorities (DoH, 1989a, para 4.20), local authorities took over responsibility for assessing and funding people entering nursing care. As Means and Smith (1998a) suggest, this has exacerbated confusion as to where the responsibility for funding and providing long-term care actually rests and may well have contributed to a situation where the division between health and social care is becoming increasing untenable (see later in this chapter and Chapter Six):

> Such a situation was bound to encourage health authorities to run down their remaining nursing-home and continuing-care bed provision. Another certainty was that some local authorities would deny they had a responsibility for some people referred to them from acute hospitals, on the grounds that their needs were essentially those of health care and not social care. The boundaries of health and social care had shifted once more, with people previously perceived as ill now being increasingly defined as having social care needs which are the responsibility of local authority and not the NHS.... This has

emerged as one of the most significant features of the health and social care reforms of the 1990s. (Means and Smith, 1998a, p 153)

Hospital discharge guidance, 1989

Also in 1989, the government issued circulars **HC(89)5** and **LAC(89)7** accompanied by a booklet entitled ***Discharge of patients from hospital*** (DoH, 1989c). These replaced a circular published 26 years previously and emphasised the need for all the agencies involved in hospital discharge to establish jointly agreed procedures (see Box 3.1 for key themes of HC[89]5). To facilitate this process, the accompanying booklet was designed to help those actually responsible for implementing the requirements of the circular, clarifying the discharge responsibilities of different professional groups. With regard to joint working and to the practicalities of discharge, the booklet emphasised a number of priorities and standards to be achieved when drawing up the required procedures:

- The procedures should provide for any necessary assessment of the patient's home circumstances to be carried out at the earliest possible stage. They should ensure that any support, help or equipment required to enable the patient or carer to cope at home is available by the time the patient leaves hospital.
- Social workers will need to be involved at an early stage, in consultation with other members of the clinical team, to ensure that appropriate and timely discharge arrangements can be made.
- The consultant and medical team should discuss with the patient the likely length of stay, the expected date of discharge and any follow-up arrangements as soon as practicable. They should also inform the patient's GP of the diagnosis, medication, the degree of patient management required and any follow-up action.
- Nursing staff should confirm the date of discharge with the patient, ensure that suitable transport arrangements have been made for the journey home and, where necessary, liaise with social services to ensure that the necessary support is provided for patients as they return home. For those living alone,

---

Box 3.1: Key themes of HC(89)5

- Discharge procedures are to be agreed with all those involved in their implementation.
- All wards and departments are to agree up-to-date discharge procedures which should be issued to all concerned.
- Procedures are to be monitored by district health authorities in collaboration with social services.
- Regional health authorities are to be informed of action taken by the end of March 1990. (Quoted in Marks, 1994, p 19)

they should also ensure that provision has been made for patients' homes to be heated and for food to be provided, that there is safe access to stairs and toilet and that it is possible to gain entry.

With hindsight it seems strange that such a circular should be issued at the same time as and with no reference to the major reforms announced in *Caring for people*. Although hospital discharge was and is a controversial issue (see later in this chapter; also, Chapter Four of this book), the publication of the circular would therefore seem to suggest a certain lack of planning and coordination at the heart of government itself.

The NHS and Community Care Act 1990

Following the publication of *Caring for people*, the implementation of the NHSCCA was delayed, and the changes were phased in over a two-year period (April 1991–April 1993):

- proposals governing the inspection of residential homes, procedures for dealing with complaints and funding for mental health services came into force from April 1991;
- community care planning became mandatory from April 1992;
- the new funding regime for community care was introduced from April 1993.

While some social services departments lamented these delays, they also provided a breathing space for the agencies involved to prepare themselves for the challenge of adapting to a new system and for the government to aid this process through further guidance.

Community care policy guidance, 1990

In 1990, the Department of Health published formal guidance, primarily addressed to social services departments and health authorities. From the very beginning, this document emphasised the importance of effective collaboration:

> Effective local collaboration is the key to making a reality of community care. All the authorities and agencies which contribute to the care of vulnerable people in their own community need to be involved in preparing and developing plans and services to meet these local needs. They need to be aware of and respect each other's roles, responsibilities and objectives and to build relationships based on this mutual understanding and respect. The interface between health and social care is a key area in planning, assessment, care management, commissioning and service delivery. Neither the White Paper nor the Act change the existing responsibilities of the NHS which will

continue to be responsible for continuous health care as outlined in the White Paper.... The objective must be to provide a service in which the boundaries between primary health care, secondary health care and social care do not form barriers seen from the perspective of the service user. (DoH, 1990, paras 1.7-9)

While the statutory responsibilities of health authorities to meet health care needs remained unchanged, the policy guidance recognised the need for agreement between health and local authorities about the services each were to provide and the criteria for admission to hospital, nursing homes and residential care. Social services departments were also to obtain health authority consent before placing users in nursing homes.

With regard to hospital admission and discharge, the guidance reiterated many of the key issues contained in the 1989 circular. While the decision to admit to, or discharge from, hospital should be taken primarily on medical grounds, it should also take account of social factors. Moreover, the decision for assessing and meeting community care needs rests with social services and local authorities should not be expected to endorse decisions about an individual's care needs taken by health authorities in advance of a recognised community care assessment. Above all, patients should not leave hospital until the supply of at least essential community care services has been agreed with them, their carers and the authorities concerned (paras 3.41-5; see also Chapter Four of this book).

Community care practice guidance, 1991

The following year saw the publication of a three-volume practice guide for health and social care practitioners and their managers (DoH/SSI, 1991a, 1991b, 1991c). The first of these, aimed at practitioners, emphasised the scope of the community care reforms to achieve a "seamless service" (DoH/SSI, 1991a, p 23) for users, based around shared values, agency agreements and valuing the contributions of different agencies. The second, aimed at managers, devotes an entire chapter to the issue of interagency arrangements, emphasising the desirability of good communication systems (both formal and informal), standard referral/assessment schedules, joint databases, mutual trust and understanding and joint training (DoH/SSI, 1991b). In particular, the guidance recognises that the implementation of the NHSCCA and changes in the nature of service provision will create challenges for the agencies involved, drawing attention to a number of key issues which may arise between health and social services. A good example of one such issue is that of hospital discharge (paras 4.50-7; see also Chapter Four of this book):

• Where discharges involve consideration of publicly funded placements in residential or nursing homes, hospital authorities have an interest in ensuring local authorities have as much notice as possible.

- Discharge plans must be agreed with patients and all the agencies involved.
- "In the event of delay or disagreement between health authorities/boards and local authorities, under no circumstances should the patient be put at risk or used as a pawn, for example, through coerced discharge home" (DoH/SSI, 1991b, para 4.53).
- Hospitals and local authorities should agree discharge procedures that are designed to cause as little delay as possible. Local authorities must ensure that they have sufficient personnel to respond to demands for assistance with discharge arrangements.

The patient's charter, 1991

Also in 1991 the Conservative government launched a *Patient's charter* (DoH, 1991) as part of a wider programme of charters designed to improve the performance of public services. While this initiative set out a wide range of standards which the NHS was expected to achieve, one of the 'key areas' identified by the government was that of hospital discharge (see also Chapter Four):

> ... before you are discharged from hospital a decision should be made about any continuing health or social care needs you may have. Your hospital will agree arrangements for meeting these needs with agencies such as community nursing services and local authority social services departments before you are discharged. You and, with your agreement, your carers will be consulted and informed at all stages. (DoH, 1991, p 15)

To ensure greater transparency, health authorities were to publish annual information about their performance against such charter standards, with the name of the person to whom patients should write with any comments.

Preparing for community care, 1992-93

As preparations continued for the implementation of the NHSCCA, there was a growing concern that arrangements were not moving quickly enough to be ready in time for the Act to come into force in April 1993. To speed up the process, a number of initiatives were developed to clarify and reinforce the policies announced in the 1989 White Paper:

- In March 1992, the Deputy Chief Executive of the NHS and the Social Services Chief Inspector published a joint letter (the *first* **Foster/Laming letter**) identifying **eight 'key tasks'** which local authorities, working closely with other agencies, must address (Box 3.2). As with later policy initiatives, the letter placed considerable emphasis on the importance of hospital discharge and continuing care arrangements (see Chapters Four and Six), reaffirming the 1989 circular (DoH, 1989c) and emphasising that neither health nor social services authorities should make unilateral withdrawals from current service or financial commitments without mutual consent (DoH, 1992a).

- A *second* **Foster/Laming letter** in September 1992 reiterated the importance of the eight key tasks and indicated a need for further progress to be made. However, the letter also contained a new requirement – that all authorities must reach agreements by 31 December 1992 on strategies governing health and local authority responsibilities for nursing home placements, estimated numbers in the first year of implementation and arrangements for integrating discharge procedures with community care assessment arrangements (DoH, 1992b). In October it was announced that evidence of these **December 31st Agreements** (as they became known) would be required before payment of the Community Care Transitional Grant (a source of money transferred from social security budgets to local authorities to help them meet their new financial commitments when the Act came into force).

- Also in September 1992, a new **Community Care Support Force** was established to disseminate good practice and assist with difficulties in implementing the community care reforms.

Box 3.2: The eight key tasks for local authorities

- Agreeing the basis for required assessment systems for individuals.
- Clarifying and agreeing arrangements for continuing care for new clients in residential and nursing care.
- Ensuring the robustness and mutual acceptability of discharge arrangements.
- Clarifying roles of GPs and primary healthcare teams.
- Ensuring that adequate purchasing and charging arrangements are in place in respect of individuals who will be receiving residential or nursing home care.
- Ensuring that financial and other management systems meet the new demands likely after 1 April 1993.
- Ensuring that staff are suitably trained, wherever appropriate on a joint basis.
- Informing the public of the arrangements made by the authority for assessment and the provision of care. (DoH, 1992b)

Hospital discharge workbook, 1994

Influenced by ongoing evidence about the patchy quality of hospital discharge (see Chapter Four), the Department of Health published a *Hospital discharge workbook* in 1994 in order to provide a framework for good practice. Although not replacing existing guidance, the workbook sought to demonstrate that good practice can be resource efficient:

> The central focus of the workbook is with the outcomes of hospital discharge, both for the individual service user, and in terms of resource effectiveness. Too often these objectives are perceived as incompatible. In fact, the workbook offers a process through which both sets of objectives can be pursued in parallel. Outcomes which are good for individuals are also a good use of resources; and the best use of resources should produce good individual outcomes. (Henwood, 1994, p 4)

Having identified the various stages and stakeholders involved in the discharge process, the workbook provides a checklist and a series of performance indicators to be used from pre-admission, through assessment, treatment, discharge and follow-up. Throughout, the emphasis is very much on the multidisciplinary nature of discharge, the potential impact of poor discharge on a range of key players and the need for effective interagency collaboration:

> The decision that a patient is medically fit for discharge can only be made by a consultant.... However, the decision to discharge a patient should be the result of a jointly agreed multidisciplinary process in which social services are responsible for assessing the needs of people for social care.... Effective hospital discharge is dependent upon the various agencies involved acknowledging their complementary responsibilities. The benefits of getting it right can include maximising individuals' chance of recovery; improved hospital bed usage; more effective targeting of scarce assessment skills, and well informed community health staff knowing exactly what contribution they need to make to the care of an individual. The costs of getting it wrong include: a poor service to patients, and unnecessarily slow recovery; GPs not knowing what has happened to their patients; social services staff receiving inappropriate referrals; disputes breaking out; unplanned re-admissions, a general wastage of resources, and the risk of bad publicity on bed blocking. The workbook focuses primarily on discharge from hospital. However, it is also apparent that a discharge from hospital is an admission – or transfer – to community care; and an admission to hospital is a transfer from the community. It is crucial, therefore, to recognise that actions and decisions made at any point in a care episode can have consequences for other parts of the health and social care system. (Henwood, 1994, p 1)

Continuing care guidance, 1995

A key feature of health and social care provision throughout the 1980s and 1990s has been the withdrawal of the NHS from the provision of long-term care. Since 1983 the number of NHS long-stay beds has reduced by 38% (a loss of 21,300 beds), with increasing numbers of NHS patients discharged to independent sector nursing and residential homes, initially funded from the social security budget and, after 1993, by social services departments (Royal Commission on Long Term Care, 1999). This has created a situation remarkably similar to that of the 1950s in which patients run the risk of falling between the eligibility criteria both of health and of social services. Described by Henwood (1992, p 28) as a "twilight zone" between health and social care, this has generated "almost a new client group, and one which is the traditional province neither of health nor of social care. These are the borderline people, the partly sick and partly well, who are perceived as too sick for residential care but not ill enough for hospital care" (1992, p 29).

Tangible evidence of this new client group was later to emerge following a report by the health service commissioner into the failure of Leeds Health Care to provide long-term care for a 55-year-old man with severe brain damage (**the 'Leeds case'**). The commissioner upheld a complaint from the patient's wife that she was being obliged to pay for nursing care which should have been provided free by the NHS. Although the commissioner's report focused specifically on the circumstances of the individual case, he also recommended that Leeds Health Care review its policy and emphasised that at the heart of the complaint was the question of where overall responsibility for continuing care lay (see Wistow, 1996; Henwood et al, 1997).

In response, the then Conservative government issued new guidance on long-term care (DoH, 1995a; see also Chapter Six). Just as circular 14/57 (MoH, 1957a) had been issued to clarify the respective roles of health and social care agencies some 40 years previously, the guidance sought to reassert the NHS's responsibilities for continuing health care. Thus, "the arrangement and funding of services to meet continuing physical and mental health care needs are an integral part of the responsibilities of the NHS. This includes, but is not limited to, the responsibility to arrange and fund an appropriate level of care from the NHS under specialist clinical supervision in hospital or in a nursing home" (DoH, 1995a, p 1).

According to the circular, health authorities and GP fundholders should continue to arrange and fund a series of services (Box 3.3). Following a multidisciplinary assessment and with regard to local eligibility criteria, the consultant should decide whether:

- the patient needs continuing inpatient care funded by the NHS. This may be as a result of ongoing, complex or unpredictable health needs, or because the patient is likely to die in the very near future;

> ## Box 3.3: Services to be arranged and funded by health authorities and GP fundholders
>
> - Specialist medical and nursing assessment.
> - Rehabilitation and recovery.
> - Palliative healthcare.
> - Continuing inpatient care under specialist supervision in hospital or in a nursing home.
> - Respite healthcare.
> - Specialist healthcare to support people in nursing homes or residential homes or the community.
> - Primary healthcare.
> - Specialist transport services. (DoH, 1995a, p 4)

- the patient needs a period of rehabilitation and recovery arranged and funded by the NHS to prepare for discharge from NHS care or to minimise the risk of discharge arrangements breaking down;
- the patient can be appropriately discharged from NHS inpatient care with either a place in a nursing/residential home funded by social services or by the patient and his or her family, or a package of health and social care to support the patient to return home.

To translate the guidance into practice, health authorities and trusts were given a strict timetable, with instructions to draw up local policies and eligibility criteria and to make arrangements to handle requests to review decisions on eligibility for continuing care by 1 April 1996. This was to take place only after local consultation, with health authorities instructed to "consult and involve fully" (DoH, 1995a, p 5) local authorities, GPs, NHS and independent sector providers and representatives of users and carers.

The importance of the implementation of the continuing care guidance was subsequently underlined by a stream of further advice, guidance, monitoring programmes and Executive Letters (DoH, 1995b, 1995c, 1995d, 1995e, 1996a, 1996b). As Henwood et al (1997, p 16-17) observe:

> The attention which was paid to the national monitoring and implementation support can be seen as an acknowledgement of the growing political concerns which have surrounded long term care, and as an indicator of the scale of the task in hand. It might also be seen as recognition of the potential which existed for local failure.

Funding for priority services, 1996

The following year, a Department of Health Executive Letter set out arrangements for targeting resources at a number of key service objectives, one of which was "tackling delayed discharge as part of the commitment to continuing care" (DoH, 1996c). To encourage a 'strategic and coherent approach', health authorities were to submit jointly agreed plans for the use of a new **Continuing Care Challenge Fund** (£16 million in 1996/97 and £20 million in 1997/98). This was designed to target initiatives which would "alleviate delays in discharge by avoiding inappropriate admissions to acute hospitals, facilitating safe discharge following effective rehabilitation and recovery, and avoiding unnecessary readmission by ensuring the availability of recovery support at home" (DoH, 1996c). Examples of relevant schemes included health services (such as 'step-down' facilities for recovery, rehabilitation schemes and increased out of hours primary care), joint services (such as home from hospital, aids and equipment and assessment pre-admission beds) and social services (such as increased domiciliary support, social care support to primary care and social care support to A&E). Proposals for access to the new fund should, among other things, be jointly agreed with social services, include a jointly agreed analysis of problems with delayed discharge and a description of existing efforts to resolve them, focus on underlying problems and bring longer-term benefits.

A new government, May 1997

Following the election of a New Labour government on 1 May 1997, the number of policy initiatives designed to achieve greater cooperation between health and social services has increased dramatically. Following its landslide victory, Labour signalled its intent to 'hit the ground running' after so long in opposition, and this is precisely what it did. Since the election there has been a raft of White Papers, Green Papers and consultation documents which seem set to revolutionise the way health and social services work together.

Winter pressures, August-October 1997

In August 1997 a letter from the Secretary of State for Health (Frank Dobson) called for "truly integrated planning and action" to reduce the pressures faced by health and social services over the winter months (DoH, 1997a). While the letter focused on short-term issues, it also recognised the need for medium- and longer-term action to prevent similar winter pressures in the future, signalling the government's determination "to help all concerned to improve their work across the boundary between community care and continuing health care". Of particular importance in reducing winter pressures was the need to ensure that hospital discharge arrangements deliver "an effective and timely outcome for patients – particularly those who need community care support". Another key feature of the letter was its emphasis on the level of cooperation between health and social services as an indication of good practice:

> Localities are making best progress where they are taking what we have called a "whole system" approach to health and social care – recognizing that the actions of any one part inevitably have consequences elsewhere. Plans and actions should acknowledge this. Passing problems across budget boundaries is not an acceptable solution to problems.

Shortly afterwards, the government announced an additional £300 million to be directed towards patient care, in part to reduce winter pressures on health and social services (DoH, 1997b). Once again, the emphasis was not only on short-term priorities, but also on the need to ensure that "the improvements in the NHS processes – including joint working with social services – brought about by this extra investment should lead to lasting changes in the pattern of care". One potential area in which the additional resources were to be spent was action to tackle delayed hospital discharges, examples of which included avoiding inappropriate admissions and readmissions, providing step-down facilities and buying nursing home places (see also Chapters Four and Five of this book).

Although this **'winter pressures' funding** was repeated in subsequent years and financed a number of innovative projects, the short-term nature of this initiative was felt by some to undermine attempts to develop longer-term solutions to current problems. More recently, the government has responded to these limitations by seeking to provide more sustained funding and by emphasising more long-term year-round planning (see, for example, DoH, 2000a, 2001a).

Better services for vulnerable people, October 1997

In October 1997, a government circular was issued to provide a medium-term agenda for services for vulnerable people (DoH, 1997c). The circular focused on three main areas:

• Health and local authorities should agree **Joint Investment Plans** for continuing and community care services. Plans were to include a joint analysis of local population needs, current resources, current investment, agreed service outcomes, agreed gaps in service provision and present and future commissioning priorities.
• Work to improve the content and process of **multidisciplinary assessment** of older people in both hospital and community health care settings. The circular recognised that existing assessments are "frequently poorly coordinated, often inappropriately timed for the patient and not targeted to those most in need. This results in a poor use of staff resources, inappropriate decisions about future care needs and a lack of equity in access to health and social care

services". To remedy this situation, health and local authorities were to review their current practice and to agree a framework for the multidisciplinary assessment of older people.
• The development of health and social care services for older people which focus on **optimising independence** through timely **recuperation** and **rehabilitation** opportunities (see Chapter Five of this book).

These issues arose during monitoring of the implementation of the 1995-96 continuing healthcare guidance. This revealed that "some health and local authorities are still not able to effectively plan their respective and joint investment in continuing and community care. They are not delivering the coordinated care that is necessary" (DoH, 1997c, annex A). A particular issue was the extent to which health and social services were working together to provide a broad safety net for those in need: "there is concern that gaps could begin to emerge between social care and health criteria as both review them in the light of resource constraints. Where local working relationships are good there is negotiation about and resolution to difficulties. Where they are not, it is a cause of significant tension". The circular also highlighted the need to update hospital discharge guidance (see Chapter Four of this book).

Special Transitional Grant, December 1997

On 5 December 1997 circular **LASSL(97)25** announced conditions for the payment of Special Transitional Grant for 1998-99 (DoH, 1997d). Particularly worthy of note was a new requirement that local authorities should use some of the grant monies allocated to them "for the purposes of preventing persons being admitted unnecessarily to hospital, or being unnecessarily placed in a residential care home or nursing home following discharge from hospital" (DoH, 1997d, annex C, para 2).

The new NHS, December 1997

Despite focusing on internal changes within the NHS, the government's 1997 White Paper placed considerable emphasis on the importance of partnership within and between health and social services (DoH, 1997e). Specific initiatives included:

• the creation of **Health Improvement Plans** (now Health Improvement and Modernisation Plans) to improve local health and healthcare. Although health authorities were to have lead responsibility for drawing up such programmes, the government pledged its commitment to establishing a new **statutory duty** for local NHS bodies to work in partnership with each other and with local authorities for the common good (paras 4.7-8);
• the setting up of pilot **Health Action Zones** from April 1998, with a series of

organisations within and beyond the NHS developing and implementing locally agreed strategies for improving the health of local people;

- a reiteration of the need for health authorities to develop **Joint Investment Plans** for continuing and community care services, first introduced under the Better Services for Vulnerable People initiative;
- provision for local authority chief executives to participate in health authority meetings;
- new evidence-based **National Service Frameworks** applicable to both health and social services to ensure consistent access to services and quality of care across the country. The first frameworks were to focus on mental health, coronary heart disease and services for older people;
- new **Primary Care Groups** (PCGs) were to bring local GPs and community nurses together in new bodies designed to improve the health of the local population. Different PCGs were to have different responsibilities, ranging from supporting the health authority in commissioning services to commissioning and providing their own primary care and community health services. In addition, each PCG was to have a social services representative on its governing body. These groups were to be piloted from April 1998, ready to 'go live' from April 1999 (see Chapter Nine of this book);
- the Department of Health committed itself to integrating policy on public health, social care and the NHS in order to provide a clear national framework. In the future, NHS Executive Regional Offices were to work with regional Social Services Inspectorates (SSIs) to monitor local action to strengthen partnerships across health and social care. A key focus was to be the extent of progress in areas such as continuing care.

In presenting the White Paper to the House of Commons, moreover, the government announced its intention to draw up a second White Paper to bring down what was described as "the Berlin Wall between health and social care" (House of Commons Debates, 1997).

Many of these policy initiatives were later reiterated in the government's **Green** and **White Papers** on **public health** (DoH, 1997f, 1999a) and implemented under the **Health Act 1999**.

Partnership in action, September 1998

In 1998, the government issued a consultation document on possible mechanisms for facilitating joint working between health and social services (DoH, 1998a). In introducing its proposals, the document provided a scathing but accurate description of the current situation and underlined the urgent need for reform:

> All too often when people have complex needs spanning both health and social care good quality services are sacrificed for sterile arguments about boundaries. When this happens people, often the most

vulnerable in our society ... and those who care for them find themselves in the no man's land between health and social services. This is not what people want or need. It places the needs of the organisation above the needs of the people they are there to serve. It is poor organisation, poor practice, poor use of taxpayers' money – it is unacceptable. (DoH, 1998a, p 3)

Despite this, the government was adamant that the solution did not lie in major organisational reforms:

> Major structural change is not the answer. We do not intend to set up new statutory health and social services authorities. They would involve new bureaucracy and would be expensive and disruptive to introduce. Our proposals set out a better course which is less bureaucratic and more efficient for users, for carers, and for staff working in those services who are often as frustrated as the people they are trying to help by the failures of the system. (DoH, 1998a, p 5)

Instead, the consultation document emphasised the need for new 'flexibilities' to remove existing barriers to joint working and enable the agencies involved to work in more collaborative and innovative ways. These included:

- **Pooled budgets:** where health and social services put a proportion of their funds into a mutually accessible joint budget. Unlike previous joint finance initiatives, contributions would lose their health or social care identity and could be used on either health or social care as appropriate. The newly created joint budget would be administered by a pool manager, supervised by a committee made up of representatives from each partner agency.
- **Lead commissioning:** where one authority transfers funds to the other which then takes responsibility for purchasing both health and social care. Services that might benefit from such an approach could be those for people with mental health problems or those with learning difficulties.
- **Integrated provision:** where one integrated organisation provides both health and social care. This would facilitate the development of more 'one stop shops' (joint premises where users can receive fast and convenient input from a number of agencies) and encourage joint training across service boundaries.

Under these proposals, authorities would be able choose to make use of these new flexibilities, notifying the Department of Health to this effect. Such powers would not be mandatory. With these new policy initiatives in place, there would be no need for previous mechanisms for collaboration such as **joint finance** or **Joint Consultative Committees** introduced in the 1970s. Whereas the former would be incorporated into health authorities' mainstream budgets, the latter would be abolished.

While the government's proposals (later confirmed in the **Health Act 1999**) were not to be introduced until April 2000, the most striking feature of the proposed changes is perhaps their similarity to the Audit Commission's proposals for a single budget for older people, lead commissioning for other user groups and the creation of community carer posts to provide more integrated services (Audit Commission, 1986). This partnership initiative has since been evaluated by researchers at the Universities of Leeds and Manchester, and the final research report provides a significant insight into partnership working under New Labour (Glendinning et al, 2002b).

Modernising social services, November 1998

Two months after the *Partnership in action* consultation document, the government introduced its eagerly awaited White Paper on social services (DoH, 1998b). In a chapter on 'Improving Partnerships', the government once again signalled its commitment to bringing down the 'Berlin Wall' between health and social services (para 6.5), but to do so in such a way as to avoid major structural reorganisation:

> Although there are often difficulties in bringing together different agencies' responsibilities, major reorganisation of service boundaries – always a tempting solution – does not provide the answer. This would simply create new boundaries and lead to instability and diversion of management effort. Instead, the government is fostering a new spirit of flexible partnership working which moves away from sterile conflicts over boundaries to an approach where this wasted time and effort is directed positively towards working across them. (DoH, 1998b, para 6.3)

To achieve this 'flexible partnership', the government reiterated and summarised the collaborative benefits to be gained from previous policies such as one stop shops, National Service Frameworks and the Winter Pressures, Better Services for Vulnerable People and Partnership in Action initiatives. However, the White Paper also contained a number of new proposals which were designed to encourage more effective joint working:

- A new **Partnership Grant** (totalling nearly £650 million over three years) was provided to foster partnership between health and social services in promoting independence as the objective of adult services. Key priorities included improving rehabilitation services, avoiding unnecessary admissions to hospital and other institutional care, improving discharge arrangements and fostering good joint contingency planning to deal with emergency pressures.

Further grants – for developing preventative services and services for carers – required action plans jointly agreed with the NHS.

- A **Fair Access to Care** initiative set out the principles authorities should follow when devising and applying eligibility criteria, including the need for compatibility with NHS continuing care criteria.
- A **Long-term Care Charter** set out at a national level what users and carers can expect if they need support from health, housing and social services.
- Regional **Commissions for Care Standards** (CCSs) were created, independent statutory bodies designed to regulate a range of domiciliary and institutional services. With health and local authority representatives on the management boards, the CCSs were to be staffed by inspectors from both health and social care backgrounds. This would bring an end to the current situation where local authorities fund nursing home care, but where responsibilities for regulation and inspection rest with health authorities. This body has since been replaced by the **Commission for Social Care Inspection**.
- There were also changes in the training and regulation of social care workers, mirroring current structures in existence in the various healthcare professions.

The Royal Commission on Long Term Care, 1999

Despite ongoing attempts to clarify responsibilities for continuing care (see earlier and Chapter Six), the provision and funding of long-term care has become an increasingly significant political issue. This was recognised from the very beginning by the New Labour government which, while in opposition, pledged its commitment to establishing a Royal Commission to investigate the matter. After the General Election, a commission was appointed in December 1997 with a brief to consider how best to fund the long-term care of older people, both in their own homes and in other settings.

When the commission presented its recommendations in March 1999, its analysis was based in part on a brutal but very accurate critique of the current funding system:

> The current system is particularly characterised by complexity and unfairness in the way it operates. It has grown up piecemeal and apparently haphazardly over the years. It contains a number of providers and funders of care, each of whom has different management or financial interests which may work against the interests of the individual client. Time and time again the letters and representations we have received from the public have expressed bewilderment with the system – how it works, what individuals should expect from it and how they can get anything worthwhile out of it. We have heard countless stories of people feeling trapped and overwhelmed by the system, and being passed from one budget to another, the consequences

sometimes being catastrophic for the individuals concerned. (Royal Commission on Long Term Care, 1999, p 33)

A key issue was the way in which the distinction between health and social care discriminates against people who have personal care needs which do not fall under the jurisdiction of the NHS. To illustrate this point further, the commission quoted the example of a person with Alzheimer's disease forced to pay for care which would be free to someone with cancer:

> Whereas the state through the NHS pays for all the care needs of sufferers from, for example cancer and heart disease, people who suffer from Alzheimer's disease may get little or no help with the cost of comparable care needs. All these conditions are debilitating, but Alzheimer's disease cannot yet be cured by medical intervention. However, a mixture of all types of care, including personal care will be needed. This is directly analogous to the kind of care provided for cancer sufferers. The latter get their care free. The former have to pay. (Royal Commission on Long Term Care, 1999, p 65)

In place of the traditional divisions between health and social care, the commission proposed a radical restructuring of the current system which would distinguish between three different types of costs:

- **living costs** (food, clothing, heating amenities and so on);
- **housing costs** (the equivalent of rent, mortgage payments and Council Tax);
- **personal care costs** (the additional cost of being looked after arising from frailty or disability).

Whereas service users would continue to pay their own housing and living costs, personal care would be free after an assessment of need and paid for by general taxation[2]. These distinctions would also be applied to domiciliary care and to aids and adaptations, with personal care services once again exempt from charges.

While the notion of free personal care has attracted the most attention, the remainder of the commission's report contained a series of proposals which will significantly affect joint working between health and social services:

- The commission suggests that the NHS has deliberately withdrawn from long-term provision in order to focus on acute care, transferring many of its costs onto social services departments. As a result, the government should analyse the shift in resources supporting long-term care since the early 1980s and consider whether there should be a transfer of resources between the NHS and social service budgets to reflect any changes in relative responsibilities.

- The commission emphasises the need for a single pooled budget for aids and adaptations.
- The commission welcomes some of the government's previous policy initiatives, supporting the introduction of Better Services for Vulnerable People, a long-term Care Charter, National Service Frameworks and the Partnership in Action proposals.
- The commission refers to the need for a single point of contact, perhaps based in primary care, for users and carers to be able to access assessment and care services.
- The commission places considerable emphasis on the potential of rehabilitation services to aid recovery and prevent the need for long-term care altogether. Despite growing awareness of the importance of rehabilitation, the commission was concerned that such services are frequently denied to people entering long-term care and vary considerably from area to area. To make rehabilitation a more integral part of service provision, the commission recommends that the value of a person's house should be disregarded for up to three months after admission to a care home, thereby providing an opportunity for recovery and convalescence before any permanent decisions need to be taken. Further research on the cost-effectiveness of rehabilitation should also be treated as a priority.

Continuing care: an ongoing issue

Following the Royal Commission's report, progress was initially slow. After an initial flurry of media attention, there was little mention of the commission's work, with some commentators suggesting that the government would rather overlook the commission's proposals altogether due to their financial implications. However, the controversies surrounding long-term care seem unlikely to go away (see Chapter Six), as evidenced by the anger and confusion generated by the case of **Pamela Coughlan**. Paralysed from the waist down after a road accident in 1971, Miss Coughlan took her local health authority to court over their attempt to close the home where she lived, transferring the patients living there from NHS to local authority services (where they might have to pay for their care). When the case came to the High Court, however, Mr Justice Hidden ruled not only that the proposed home closure was unlawful, but also that all nursing care is the responsibility of the NHS and should not be transferred onto social services. This was greeted with enthusiasm by user groups and professional organisations, who felt that it would lead to the provision of free nursing home care and prevent the NHS from shifting its responsibilities for continuing care onto social services (Dyer, 1998; Shaw, 1998):

> Nursing is 'health care' and can never be 'social care'. (Quoted in Shaw, 1998).

Aided by the Department of Health, the health authority immediately appealed and a judgement from the Appeal Court was announced in July 1999. While the Appeal Court ruled that the proposed home closure was unlawful, it did not back the previous judgement that nursing care should be provided by the NHS rather than social services. This has generated a series of conflicting interpretations, with some commentators claiming that the judgement will end means-testing for nursing care and others arguing that social services remain responsible for funding such services (Hunter, 1999). The Health Secretary (Frank Dobson) was apparently "delighted", stressing that the Appeal Court's decision confirms the role of social services in arranging nursing home care (DoH, 1999b). In response, the government promised to review continuing care policy in light of the judgement, issuing interim guidance until a review could be carried out (DoH, 1999c). Following the Coughlan case, health and local authorities, in consultation with each other, should "satisfy themselves that their continuing and community care policies and eligibility criteria and other relevant procedures are in line with the judgment and existing guidance, taking further legal advice where necessary". Above all, they must "work together in partnership to ensure that service users do not fall between 'gaps' in services" (DoH, 1999c, p 3).

In particular, the Coughlan judgement emphasised that the decision as to whether or not someone should receive free NHS continuing care depended on whether or not the nursing services concerned are:

- merely incidental or ancillary to the provision of accommodation which a local authority is under duty to provide;
- of a nature which it could not be expected that an authority whose primary responsibility is to provide social services could be expected to provide (quoted in DoH, 2001b; Health Service Ombudsman, 2003).

More recently, these developments have been summarised in a **new continuing care circular** (DoH, 2001b), which seeks to consolidate previous guidance in light of the Coughlan judgement, ensure that the NHS and local councils agree together how they will meet continuing health and social care needs and update the review and complaints procedures for continuing care. Unfortunately, all the available evidence suggests that the complexity which characterises long-term care policy will continue, with accusations by the **Health Service Ombudsman** (2003) that local NHS bodies are using overly restrictive eligibility criteria for continuing care which are not in line with the Coughlan judgement or Department of Health guidance.

Overall, the Ombudsman concludes that:

> Any [funding] system [for long-term care] must be fair and logical and should be transparent in respect of the entitlement of individuals. From what I have seen, the national policy and guidance that has been in place over recent years does not pass that test. Those who

complain to me find the system far from fair or logical and often cannot understand why they or a relative are not entitled to NHS funding. At times entitlement seems to have depended in part variously on ill-defined distinctions between:

- specialist and general health care;
- health care and social care;
- care by registered nurses and care by others.

The distinction between health and social care ... is a blurred one which has ... shifted over time.... Some patients needing long term care might need help with a wide range of basic activities: to the average patient or carer, the distinction professionals might make between health and social needs is largely irrelevant. (Health Service Ombudsman, 2003, pp 6-7)

As a result of this chain of events, strategic health authorities are now responsible for establishing a single set of continuing care criteria in all the PCTs in their area and money is being set aside to reimburse those older people incorrectly charged for care they should have received free (for the latest developments, visit www.dh.gov.uk).

The government's response to the Royal Commission, 2000

While controversy was continuing to rage over the Coughlan case and its potential implications, the government published its response to the Royal Commission in July 2000 (DoH, 2000b). In accepting the vast majority of the commission's recommendations, the government also acknowledged the importance of partnership working between health, social care and housing in meeting the needs of older people:

Stronger and deeper partnerships between health and social care agencies will be needed in many places, with better communications, pooling of budgets and more integrated services. They should also bring in housing agencies to provide a greater choice of suitable accommodation. (DoH, 2000b, p 5)

One example of the government's commitment to partnership working is the pledge to create **integrated community equipment stores** by March 2004 (see DoH, 2001c, 2001d, 2001e, 2001f for further details).

Despite its support for most of the commission's recommendations, however, the government rejected the central plank of the commission's report: the call for free personal care. Although making personal care free would cost a substantial sum of money, the government argued, it would merely shift the cost of such services from the individual to the state, without necessarily improving those services or leading to any increases in the overall amount of money invested in such provision at all. Instead, the government pledged to introduce **free NHS nursing care**, so that the costs of "registered nurse time spent on providing, delegating or supervising care" would be free to everyone who needs it, whether they live at home, in residential care or in a nursing home (DoH, 2000b, p 11) from October 2001. This meant that older people in residential or nursing care would continue to pay for their personal care and accommodation costs as before:

> There can be no justification for charging people in care homes for their nursing costs. We will make nursing care available free under the NHS to everyone in a care home who needs it.... This change will benefit around 35,000 people at any time. They could save up to around £5,000 for a year's stay in a nursing home. The introduction of free nursing care in every setting will provide the right incentives to the NHS and social services to work together to provide the modern quality care that people need. It will encourage the NHS to provide rehabilitation services that people are able to benefit from. It will reduce the perverse incentive to discharge people too early to social services funded care. It will create a fairer system, where people can receive the nursing care they need wherever they live, paid for or provided by the NHS. It will end the most obvious inconsistency in the funding of long term care. (DoH, 2000b, pp 11-12)

This proposal was subsequently introduced under section 49 of the **Health and Social Care Act 2001**, and further guidance has been issued to clarify and amend the government's initial pledge (see, for example, DoH, 2001g, 2003a). In the event, free nursing care was only introduced for people paying the full cost of their care ('self-funders') as of 1 October 2001, with local authority-supported residents in nursing homes receiving NHS-funded nursing care from April 2003. Under this system, the NHS will pay for the costs of registered nursing time following an assessment of individuals' needs by a NHS nurse (using an assessment tool known as the **Registered Nursing Care Contribution** or RNCC). Fees will then be paid to the nursing home concerned according to one of three bands:

- *low* (£40 per week from 1 April 2003);
- *medium* (£75 per week);
- *high* (£120 per week).

To finance this new system, funds previously spent by local councils on nursing care are being reallocated to the NHS to help meet its new commitments.

Interestingly, a different policy has been adopted in **Scotland**, which is following the recommendation of the Royal Commission to implement free personal care (see, for example, Care Development Group, 2001; Royal Commission on Long Term Care, 2003). Over time, it is possible that this may place increased pressure on Whitehall to follow suit, and certainly gives a very strong example of the potential that devolution has to develop different policy responses in different parts of the UK.

Also rejected by the government was the Royal Commission's proposal to examine the shift in resources between health and social care and to transfer funding to social services if local authorities were found to have taken on additional responsibilities from the NHS. This was deemed not to be necessary in light of a significant growth in partnership working between health and social care, which presumably was felt to make such an exercise overly controversial and ultimately counter-productive. Whether or not the government felt that such a shift in responsibilities had occurred without a transfer of adequate funding was not stated.

The NHS plan, 2000

In the event, the government's response to the Royal Commission was almost entirely overshadowed by a new policy initiative launched at the same time. In July 2000, *The NHS plan* set out the government's long-term vision for the NHS (DoH, 2000c). Described by the Prime Minister as "historic" and "radical" (DoH, 2000c, pp 8-9), the plan covered a wide range of issues from funding to staff recruitment and retention, from NHS buildings to patient-centred care and from relationships with the private sector to reductions in waiting times for treatment. However, a four-page chapter (in a 144-page document) focused on 'Changes between health and social services', launching a number of potentially significant new policies. An additional chapter focused in more detail on 'Dignity, security and independence in old age'. Overall, the government emphasised that substantial change was required:

> If patients are to receive the best care, then the old divisions between health and social care need to be overcome. The NHS and social services do not always work effectively together as partners in care, so denying patients access to seamless services that are tailored to their particular needs. The division between health and social services can often be a source of confusion for people. Fundamental reforms are needed to tackle these problems. (DoH, 2000c, p 70)

Key initiatives included:

- Greater emphasis on the **co-location** of health and social care services (for example, in GP surgeries).
- A promise to make all areas of the country use the **'flexibilities'** introduced under the Health Act 1999.

49

- An extra £900 million investment by 2003/04 in new **intermediate care** services to promote independence through active recovery and rehabilitation services, prevent unnecessary admission to hospital and enable more people to live independently at home (see Chapter Five of this book). Designed to provide "the right care at the right time in the right place" (DoH, 2000c, p 71), intermediate care might include:
  - ▸ multidisciplinary rapid response teams to care for people at home and prevent unnecessary hospital admissions;
  - ▸ intensive rehabilitation services to help older people regain their independence after a stroke or major surgery;
  - ▸ recuperation facilities in nursing homes;
  - ▸ one-stop services in primary care;
  - ▸ integrated home care teams to facilitate swift hospital discharges.
- **Joint inspections** of health and social care organisations (using the Best Value system) by the Commission for Health Improvement, Audit Commission and the SSI.
- A new **National Performance Fund** to make incentive payments to encourage and reward joint working.
- The transition of all PCGs into **Primary Care Trusts (PCTs)** by April 2004 (see Chapter Nine of this book). Whereas PCGs were sub-committees of the health authority with devolved responsibility for the healthcare needs of their local community, PCTs are free-standing, legally established statutory NHS bodies. According to *The NHS plan*, this move from PCGs to PCTs has the potential to improve partnership working between health and social care as these new organisations have the potential to make "the health and social care system easier to understand, simpler to access and more convenient to use" (DoH, 2000c, p 73). Quite how these changes were to occur from the transition to PCT status was not set out.
- A new type of organisation (a **Care Trust**) based on the PCT model to commission and deliver health and social care. At this stage, the detail on what a Care Trust might look like or do was very sparse, and this new way of working was introduced in four brief paragraphs:

> We now propose to establish a new level of primary care trusts which will provide for even closer integration of health and social services. In some parts of the country, health and social services are already working together extremely closely and wish to establish new single multi-purpose legal bodies to commission and be responsible for all local health and social care. The Government intends to build on the establishment of primary care trusts so that all those localities who want to follow this route can do so. This will require changes to the governance arrangements for primary care trusts to ensure representation of health and social care partners. The new body will be known as a 'Care Trust' to reflect its new broader role.

Care Trusts will be able to commission and deliver primary and community healthcare as well as social care for older people and other client groups. Social services would be delivered under delegated authority from local councils. Care Trusts will usually be established where there is a joint agreement at local level that this model offers the best way to deliver better care services.

Where local health and social care organisations have failed to establish effective joint partnerships – or where inspection or joint reviews have shown that services are failing – the Government will take powers to establish integrated arrangements through the new Care Trust.

The establishment of Care Trusts will obviously have to take account of the roll out and capacity of primary care trusts. The first wave of Care Trusts could be in place next year [2001]. (DoH, 2000c, p 73)

- A **single assessment process** for health and social care.
- A **personal care plan** for older people setting out their health and social care package.
- A new service (**Care Direct**) to provide information and advice about health, social care, housing, pensions and benefits by telephone, drop-in centres, online and through outreach services.
- A new *National service framework for older people* to set out clear standards for older people's services (including both health and social care).

Since the publication of *The NHS plan*, many of these initiatives have been developed substantially in further guidance and official documents. Of particular significance are the following four policies:

1. Intermediate care has since been defined in greater detail in the *National service framework for older people* (see later in this chapter) and a government circular (DoH, 2001e, 2001f; see also Chapter Five of this book). Essentially, intermediate care is designed to prevent unnecessary hospital admissions, facilitate swift and timely hospital discharges and prevent premature admissions to permanent residential and nursing care. According to **circular 2001/001**, intermediate care should be regarded as describing services that meet *all* the following criteria (DoH, 2001e, p 6):

   - are targeted at people who would otherwise face unnecessarily prolonged hospital stays or inappropriate admission to acute inpatient care, long-term residential care, or continuing NHS inpatient care;
   - are provided on the basis of a comprehensive assessment, resulting in a structured individual care plan that involves active therapy, treatment or opportunity for recovery;

- have a planned outcome of maximising independence and typically enabling patients/users to resume living at home;
- are time-limited, normally no longer than six weeks and frequently as little as one to two weeks or less;
- involve cross-professional working, with a single assessment framework, single professional records and shared protocols.

In order to offer users and carers a seamless service, the NHS and councils should make optimum use of pooled budgets, other Health Act flexibilities and the developing Care Trust model. Intermediate care services should also be provided to patients free of charge and should generally be located in community-based settings or in the patient's own home. The NHS and councils should ensure that systems for evaluating intermediate care services are built in from the earliest possible stage of planning and implementation. They should also consult and take into account the views of patients/users and carers on current patterns of service delivery and on the potential impact of developing new intermediate care services. Throughout, the NHS and local authorities should take into account the potential contribution of the independent sector and, where appropriate, develop services in partnership with independent providers (see Chapter Five of this book for further information).

2. Local NHS and social care organisations are working to introduce a **single assessment process** for older people by April 2004. Subsequent government guidance and documentation has specified that local health and social care organisations should base local assessment mechanisms on four different levels of assessment (DoH, 2001h):

- contact assessment (information collected on the presenting problem at the first contact with formal services);
- overview assessment (carried out if the professional feels that the person needs a more rounded assessment);
- specialist assessments (to explore specific needs);
- comprehensive assessment (where prolonged/intensive support is likely to be required or where the person requires specialist assessments across a range of areas).

Once an assessment is completed, information should be stored in a systematic way and shared between health and social care agencies so as to prevent service users and carers from having to supply the same information to different professionals.

3. The Care Trust model has been formally introduced under the **Health and Social Care Act 2001**. At the time of writing, there are eight Care Trusts in England – five focusing on mental health and based on previous NHS provider

trusts, and three based on primary care organisations, commissioning as well as providing services. In the event, the government's desire to compel failing local agencies to form Care Trusts was not included in the legislation, and the model remains a voluntary one. For further information, see Glasby and Peck's (2003) *Care trusts* or visit the Department of Health website (see, for example, DoH, 2001i).

4. The transition from PCGs to PCTs was accelerated under the **Shifting the balance of power** initiative (DoH, 2001j). As a result, all remaining PCGs became PCTS (or Care Trusts) by April 2002, and are now the lead NHS organisation in assessing need, planning and securing all health services and improving health. They are also the NHS body with the most scope to work in partnership with local authorities (including social services departments). As part of the same policy initiative, the 95 former health authorities have been replaced with a much smaller number (28) of strategic health authorities. Although these changes will impact primarily on the NHS, the subsequent reorganisation of the NHS has meant that primary care is now the main arena for partnership working between health and social care (see Chapter Nine for further discussion).

The National service framework for older people, 2001

In March 2001, the *National service framework for older people* (DoH, 2001f) provided a long-term vision of the future of services for older people and set a series of national standards to improve quality and reduce variations in care in different areas of the country. The third such framework to be produced by New Labour, it is based on four key principles:

- respecting the individual;
- promoting intermediate care;
- providing evidence-based specialist care;
- promoting an active, healthy life.

In order to implement these principles, the framework sets out a series of eight service standards (each of which include a series of key interventions that will be required and a number of milestones that will need to be met) (Box 3.4).

Delivering the NHS plan, 2002

In April 2002, **Delivering the NHS plan** (DoH, 2002b) described the steps which have been taken to begin to deliver on the commitments of *The NHS plan* and additional actions that are required to make further progress. In a three-page chapter on health and social care, the document summarises many of the earlier policies and suggests the need for further change (see page 55).

Box 3.4: The *National service framework for older people*

Standard 1: Rooting out age discrimination – NHS services will be provided, regardless of age, on the basis of clinical need alone. Social care services will not use age in their eligibility criteria or policies, to restrict access to available services.

Standard 2: Person-centred care – NHS and social care services treat older people as individuals and enable them to make choices about their own care. This is achieved through the single assessment process, integrated commissioning arrangements and integrated provision of services, including community equipment and continence services.

Standard 3: Intermediate care – older people will have access to a new range of intermediate care services at home or in designated care settings, to promote their independence by providing enhanced services from the NHS and councils to prevent unnecessary hospital admission and effective rehabilitation services to enable early discharge from hospital and to prevent premature or unnecessary admission to long-term residential care (see Chapter Five of this book for further discussion).

Standard 4: General hospital care – older people's care in hospital is delivered through appropriate specialist care and by hospital staff who have the right set of skills to meet their needs (see Chapter Four for discussion of hospital discharge).

Standard 5: Stroke – the NHS will take action to prevent strokes, working in partnership with other agencies where appropriate. People who are thought to have had a stroke have access to diagnostic services, are treated appropriately by a specialist stroke service, and subsequently, with their carers, participate in a multidisciplinary programme of secondary prevention and rehabilitation.

Standard 6: Falls – the NHS, working in partnership with councils, takes action to prevent falls and reduce resultant fractures or other injuries in their populations of older people. Older people who have fallen receive effective treatment and rehabilitation and, with their carers, receive advice on prevention through a specialised falls service.

Standard 7: Mental health in older people – older people who have mental health problems have access to integrated mental health services, provided by the NHS and councils to ensure effective diagnosis, treatment and support, for them and for their carers (see Chapter Eight of this book for further discussion).

Standard 8: The promotion of health and active life in older age – the health and well-being of older people is promoted through a coordinated programme of action led by the NHS with support from councils. (DoH, 2001f)

Although progress has been made towards breaching the 'Berlin Wall' between health and social care there are still too many parts of the country where a failure to cooperate means that older people fail to get the holistic services they need. Older people are the single biggest users of the NHS. They are the generation which built and have supported the NHS all their lives. The commitment to deliver patient-centred care – the right care, in the right place, at the right time – must, above all, be honoured in the delivery of care for older people. And older people above all others have a right to expect that their care is delivered seamlessly through a range of services that are convenient and as close to home as possible. (DoH, 2002b, p 32)

To deliver this seamless provision, the document outlines a number of potential developments, including:

- new measures to prevent delayed hospital discharges (see later in this chapter and Chapter Four);
- financial incentives to encourage the voluntary take-up of Care Trust status;
- additional (as yet unspecified) incentives to encourage closer integration of health and social care.

However, *Delivering the NHS plan* concludes with a relatively dramatic summary that seems to leave the way open for further reform in the future and suggests that the boundary between health and social care might be the subject of further, possibly radical, action:

Finally, we will keep the relationship between health and social services under review. Older people and other service users have the right to expect that local services are working as one care system not two. We will monitor how far the NHS Plan and these further reforms we are proposing take us towards that goal. If more radical change is needed we will introduce it. (DoH, 2002b, p 33)

Hospital discharge: an ongoing issue

Throughout New Labour's time in office, the issue of delayed hospital discharges has become an increasingly significant issue (see also Chapter Four of this book). According to former Health Secretary, Alan Milburn (DoH, 2001k):

Bed-blocking is a major problem for all NHS patients. Bed-blocking leaves people in beds who should be cared for elsewhere and keeps people from beds who need treatment straight away. We are determined to tackle this problem which has bedevilled the health service for decades so that patients receive the right care in the right place at the right time.

Since May 1997, key policy initiatives have included (see Glasby, 2003a for an overview):

- A £300 million **'Cash for Change'** initiative to reduce the number of delayed discharges (DoH, 2001k). This has since been linked to a new **Concordat** or agreement between the public and independent sectors (DoH, 2001l). More recently, this has been replaced by a new **Access and Systems Capacity Grant** to fund home improvement services, purchase community equipment and improve home care and intermediate care services (DoH, 2003b).
- The creation in January 2002 of the **Health and Social Care Change Agent Team** to support the implementation of the *National service framework for older people*, to develop a single system of health and social care and to work with local agencies to reduce delayed hospital discharges (DoH, 2003c).
- A **House of Commons Health Committee** (2002) inquiry into delayed hospital discharges and a report by the **National Audit Office** (2003).
- The publication of a new *Discharge from hospital* **workbook** (DoH, 2003d) to replace the 1994 predecessor described earlier. Emphasising the need for a whole systems approach, the workbook covers a wide range of topics, from user involvement to continuing care and from coordinating the patient journey to the role of housing services.

Above all, however, the key measure has been the introduction of new legislation (**The Community Care [Delayed Discharges etc] Act 2003**) to charge social services departments for hospital beds unnecessarily 'blocked' by people awaiting social services provision (Box 3.5). As the Department of Health (2002b, p 33, emphasis added) explains:

> We have been impressed by the success of the system in countries like Sweden and Denmark in getting delayed discharges from hospitals down. We intend to legislate therefore to introduce a similar system of **cross-charging** [also known as **'reimbursement'**]. The new social services cash announced in the Budget includes resources to cover the cost of beds needlessly blocked in hospitals through delayed discharges.... Councils will need to use these extra resources to expand care at home and to ensure that all older people are able to leave hospital once their treatment is completed and it is safe for them to do so. If councils reduce the number of blocked beds, they will have the freedom to use these new resources to invest in alternative social care services. If they cannot meet the agreed time limit they will be charged by the local hospital for the costs it incurs in keeping older people in hospital unnecessarily. In this way there will be far

stronger incentives in the system to ensure that patients do not have to experience long delays in their discharge from hospital. There will be matching incentive charges on NHS hospitals to make them responsible for the costs of emergency hospital readmissions, so as to ensure patients are not discharged prematurely.

At the time of writing, it is still too early to tell exactly how this new measure will work in practice, although it has certainly aroused considerable controversy and criticisms from a range of commentators (see, for example, Clode, 2002; Glasby, 2002a, 2002b; Glendinning, 2002). Perhaps the highest profile of these critics has been the House of Commons Health Committee (2002), which stressed

Box 3.5: Reimbursement

The Government announced its intention to introduce a system of reimbursement in *Delivering the NHS plan* in April 2002. It is based on a system used in Scandinavia that has had a major impact on reducing delayed discharges.

The Community Care (Delayed Discharges etc.) Bill was introduced into the House of Commons on 14 November 2002. The Bill received Royal Assent on 8 April 2003....

This Act aims to improve and strengthen discharge planning and the timely provision of the services patients need to transfer from one care setting to another....

The Act places certain duties on NHS organizations and councils:

- NHS bodies have a new statutory duty to notify social services of a patient's 'likely need for community care services'... and their proposed discharge date....

- There is then a defined timescale for social services to complete the individual's assessment and provide appropriate social care services [a minimum of two days is set out in the Act].

- A reimbursement charge of £100/120 per day [£100 per day for most departments, but £120 for London and the South East] is paid by social services to the acute trust if the fact of social services not having met their obligations – that is, to assess the patient (and carer if appropriate) and provide social care services within the set time – is the *sole* reason for the delay in discharge from hospital. If any element of the delay is related to NHS areas of responsibility then reimbursement does not apply. (DoH, 2003e, pp 3-6) the potential of the new Act to lead to "an unproductive culture of buck passing and mutual blame" (2002, p 52; see Chapter Four of this book for further discussion). However, one potential advantage of the new scheme is that hospitals will be obliged to **assess patients for continuing care** before notifying social services of a potential discharge.

Summary

While the policy and legal context is constantly changing, this overview of key health and social care policy initiatives suggests a number of overriding themes and issues which have tended to characterise official responses to partnership working and interagency collaboration over a long period of time. In particular:

- There is a tendency for government policy to exhort frontline workers and agencies to work more effectively together. Using the framework of individual, organisational and structural levels of activity set out in Chapter Two of this book, interventions have often been at the I and O level, rather than at a national level. At different times in our recent history, this has left health and social care agencies (and those who work in them) trying to collaborate more effectively with partners from different professional and organisational backgrounds without adequate government action to remove the administrative, legal and bureaucratic barriers that have bedevilled all previous attempts to work in partnership (see Glasby, 2003a, for a further discussion).
- The boundary between health and social care has shifted considerably over time, with more and more areas of service provision that would once have been defined as 'healthcare' falling under the remit of local authority social services departments. Thus, local authority care homes for people during minor illness and for 'infirm' residents in the late 1950s have been gradually transformed into much more specialist services caring for people with much greater health and social care needs than would ever once have been the case. Of course, this has significant implications for users and carers (as healthcare tends to be free at the point of delivery, while social care can attract substantial user charges). Despite the recommendation of the Royal Commission on Long Term Care that these shifts in the boundary between health and social care should be examined and resources reallocated as appropriate, the New Labour government has decided not to pursue this issue.
- Sometimes, the same themes and issues have emerged time and time again in different contexts and in response to slightly different circumstances. Examples include the similarities between the Audit Committee and Select Committee reports of the mid-1980s and the Health Act flexibilities of 1999, ongoing difficulties associated with delayed hospital discharges and a lack of clarity about responsibility for long-term and continuing care from the 1950s to the 21st century.

- In recent years, there has been a noticeable shift from discretionary and enabling policies (such as the Health Act flexibilities or winter pressures funding) to an approach based more on compulsion and/or punitive measures (such as the desire to compel agencies to form Care Trusts, reimbursement or the tone of *Delivering the NHS plan*). At the same time, the belief in the need to avoid major restructuring of health and social care set out in the *Partnership in action* discussion document appears to have been replaced with more of an emphasis on reorganisation and potentially radical action (as expressed in *Shifting the balance of power* and *Delivering the NHS plan*). Quite what this means for the future is currently unclear, but it seems unlikely that the current policy context will remain as it is for long, and further change may be imminent.

Above all, however, this chapter gives an example of the complexity of health and social care policy. In summarising key developments, we have only included a fraction of the vast array of policy documents, statutes and consultations that have been produced, and even this brief overview has, at times, proved long and complicated. If this is what the system feels like to policy makers, social policy analysts, students and frontline workers, then what must it be like for older people who use the services concerned or their carers? It is to this that we turn in Chapters Four to Nine.

Notes

[1] Although commentators usually focus solely on the contents of *Caring for people*, it should be noted that this publication was accompanied by a second White Paper, *Working for patients*, which concentrated primarily on internal changes within the health services (DoH, 1989b).

[2] The notion of free personal care was not uncontested, and two members of the commission submitted an additional report contained at the end of the commission's main findings arguing for the need to means-test personal care.

Further reading

While individual policy documents can often be obtained in hard copy format or via the Department of Health website (www.dh.gov.uk), it can be very difficult to keep up to date with changes in health and social care policy. Accessible chronologies such as that provided in this chapter are unfortunately relatively rare, and readers wishing to keep abreast of the latest developments are recommended to consult the following sources:

- Practitioner- and manager-focused magazines (such as *Community Care, Nursing Older People* and the *Health Service Journal*).

- The 'What's new on the site?' section of www.dh.gov.uk.

- The Tertiary Care section of the Department of Health's website (www.dh.gov.uk/PolicyAndGuidance/OrganisationPolicy/TertiaryCare).

- Professional associations (such as the Association of Directors of Social Services, the Royal Colleges and the NHS Confederation).

- Voluntary organisations (such as Age Concern or Help the Aged).

For background material on the history of health and social care, the work of Means and Smith provides an excellent and accessible overview (Means and Smith, 1998b; Means et al, 2002). Also useful is Lewis' (2001) overview of the health–social care divide in services for older people. Bradley and Manthorpe (2000) also offer a summary of the problematic nature of the health–social care divide, citing a series of practical examples and research studies to illustrate the issues at stake.

FOUR

Andrew's story: hospital discharge

For service users and professionals alike, the ability of health and social services to ensure the efficient and effective discharge of patients from hospital is often an acid test of how well these two agencies are working together. More than any other issue, that of hospital discharge is fundamental to the experience of working at the interface between health and social services and to the quality of care provided. After a review of recent research findings, this chapter tells the story of Andrew, a man whose experience of hospital discharge was far removed from the 'seamless service' so strongly emphasised during the community care reforms.

Exercise F: Hospital discharge

Before reading this chapter, consider:

1. How might an older person in hospital be feeling about the possibility of being discharged from hospital?
2. How might their family be feeling?
3. Are there particular situations or services where the responsibilities of health and social care could overlap?
4. If so, what steps could practitioners and services take to ensure that the services offered to older people are as coordinated as possible?
5. Which of the policies in Chapter Three might help to achieve this goal?

Research findings and service issues

In recent years, the discharge of older people from hospital has received considerable attention from policy makers (see Chapter Three), professional bodies (BGS/ADSS/RCN, 1995) and researchers (Neill and Williams, 1992; Henwood and Wistow, 1993; Marks, 1994; Phillipson and Williams, 1995). It is now recognised that hospital discharge can be a major life event for both patient and carer, with significant implications for the best use of scarce health and social care resources (Henwood, 1994). In response, a series of attempts has been made at both a national and a local level to ensure that hospital discharges proceed in a planned, coordinated way which achieves a 'seamless' service in which the patient experiences a continuity of health and social care (DoH, 1990; DoH/SSI, 1991a). Despite this, research reveals that success has thus far been elusive.

For example, in 1992, a National Institute of Social Work study of hospital discharge and older people in four local authority areas found that one in five participants had a very poor discharge, with only one in three experiencing a good discharge (Neill and Williams, 1992). This assessment was made on the basis that a 'good' hospital discharge occurs when the older person:

- is given at least 24 hours' notice of discharge;
- is given an opportunity to discuss how they would manage after discharge;
- has somebody with them on the journey home;
- has somebody waiting for them at home;
- has somebody who calls to see them on the day of discharge (Neill and Williams, 1992, p 82).

More specifically, the study found evidence of poor collaborative practice, a lack of communication and a failure to implement the requirements of the 1989 hospital discharge guidance (DoH, 1989c):

- Links between hospital and GPs were weak and only one in three wards routinely gave patients written information about their medication.
- Relationships between social workers and hospital staff were very variable, ranging from serious conflict to good collaboration. Key issues included unrealistic expectations of each other's role and disagreements between managers over resources and procedures.
- Most referrals for home help services were received on the day of discharge or after the patient had left hospital. Only half the people referred were considered by the home help organisers to actually need this service.
- One quarter of patients felt they had been discharged too soon and one third had no discussion with staff about how they would manage at home. Two fifths were given one day's notice or less.
- On the day of discharge itself, patients found waiting for transport exhausting and there was little consideration of how they would manage getting from hospital transport to their homes. Seventeen per cent arrived home on their own and were alone for the rest of the day. While many people had someone to prepare their house for them, others came back to unheated homes, with food that had gone bad, dead houseplants and dust. While major items of equipment were usually provided on or soon after the day of discharge, patients could wait weeks or even months for some aids and adaptations.
- Two weeks after discharge nearly all the sample could be described as severely disabled, most lacked some self-care ability, two thirds were experiencing some degree of pain, three quarters described poor sleeping patterns, three fifths described some loss of bladder control and one in three were possibly clinically depressed. Only one in four said they felt well.

In summing up, the researchers highlighted the plight of a small number of older service users "who are at the sensitive interface between residential care, readmission to hospital and care in the community" (DoH, 1989c, p 157). These people usually required more support than current services were able to provide, prompting the researchers to conclude that "this is a key group as far as the NHSCCA is concerned, and their experience provides a measure by which the success or failure of the Act may be judged" (p 157). The findings of this study were later disseminated to health and social care practitioners through a series of workshops, where participants were invited to identify and implement actions to improve the hospital discharge process (Phillipson and Williams, 1995).

In 1993, a study of hospital discharge arrangements in six English localities once again highlighted the problematic nature of the health and social care divide (Henwood and Wistow, 1993). Although policies were in an evolutionary state following the implementation of the NHS Community Care Act (NHSCCA), the authors of the research identified a fundamental tension between two competing notions of good practice in health and social services. On the one hand, there is a narrowly defined resource management model which seeks to make cost-effective use of scarce resources and to maximise the throughput of patients. On the other hand, there is the user-centred care management model which emphasises choice and needs-led assessment. Nowhere is this more clearly illustrated than in debates about so-called 'bed blocking' by patients, often older people, who have been declared medically fit for discharge, but for one reason or another cannot or will not leave hospital (Box 4.1).

Box 4.1: 'Bed blocking'

Typically associated with frail and isolated older people, the term 'bed blocking' is often used to refer to patients who are occupying a hospital bed when they do not require the services provided there, yet (for whatever reason) cannot be discharged. As Victor (1997, p 103) has observed, however, "such patients are inevitably given the highly pejorative label 'bed blockers' which implies that it is the older person's fault that they cannot be discharged. This is highly inaccurate as it is almost always the case that people cannot be discharged because we cannot supply the appropriate services for them. People who fall into this category are at the interface of the health and social care systems and often experience prolonged stays in hospital because of the difficulties the two systems experience in organizing 'seamless' care across this administrative divide". This has since been recognised by the Department of Health and the House of Commons Health Committee, and terms such as 'delayed discharges' or 'delayed transfers of care' are now felt to be more appropriate (see Glasby, 2003a, for further discussion).

Although the issue of 'bed blocking' has acquired a new impetus following the introduction of the NHSCCA, it is by no means a new problem and has been highlighted as a potential concern ever since the 1940s. As a result, a number of studies have sought to identify the number of patients inappropriately occupying hospital beds, with estimates ranging from 4.8% in Liverpool (Rubin and Davies, 1975) to 13% in east London (Murphy, 1977) and 14% in Bromley (Coid and Crome, 1986), but reaching as high as 45% days of care (Smith et al, 1997) and 62% bed days (Anderson et al, 1988) in more recent studies using more objective methods of assessment.

Despite this preoccupation with the issue of blocked beds, research has suggested that delayed discharges frequently occur for reasons beyond the control of either the health or social care workers involved (Roberts and Houghton, 1996). Moreover, the extent to which attention is focused on 'bed blocking' can also be seen as an acid test of the state of working relations between health and social services, associated more with attempts to shift blame to other agencies than with genuine attempts to resolve difficult situations through collaborative work (Henwood et al, 1997). While the term 'bed blocking' is still widely used, therefore, it masks a much more complex reality.

In 1994, a literature review published by The King's Fund Institute drew attention once again to the problematic nature of many hospital discharges, likening them to a 'patchwork quilt' rather than the 'seamless care' envisaged by government (Marks, 1994). Drawing on studies dating back more than 20 years, Marks highlights the ongoing failure to develop coherent discharge policies and practices which contrast strongly with countries like the US (where differences in the nature and funding of healthcare have increasingly focused attention on discharge as a discrete and important process). Key issues have included:

- Poor discharges, with inadequate planning, insufficient notice for patients and delays in providing community services.
- Concerns to ensure the cost-effective use of acute hospital beds by taking action to prevent 'bed blocking', reducing the length of hospital stays and discharging patients with greater health needs.
- Poor communication and a lack of collaboration between health and social services.

In 1997, the Nuffield Institute for Health published the results of its hospital discharge sub-study, carried out as part of a wider piece of research on interagency collaboration (Henwood et al, 1997). The study found that hospital discharge was still a matter of continuing difficulty in all of the six localities investigated, with patchy implementation of agreed discharge arrangements and recognised deficiencies in communication and coordination within and between agencies. Particular issues included:

- Different professional backgrounds, priorities and values. In particular, respondents drew a distinction between geriatric wards (where multidisciplinary working was more established) and medical and surgical wards (where discharges were faster, more pressurised and more hierarchical).
- Ongoing concerns with 'bed blocking', particularly under conditions of resource constraint or at times of particular pressure. Often, this was the result of a much more fundamental issue: the different models of good practice first identified earlier by Henwood and Wistow (1993).
- The increasing complexity of discharge as a result of reductions in the length of patient stays.
- Poor communication and coordination.
- A temptation to shunt costs to other agencies as a result of resource pressures.
- Difficulties identifying where and why problems were arising as a result of shortcomings in monitoring information.

A further contribution to the growing body of research on hospital discharge has come from the Social Services Inspectorate (SSI). In 1995, a study of the arrangements made by seven social services departments for the discharge of older people from hospital to residential or nursing home care highlighted a number of key issues (DoH/SSI, 1995a). Despite making considerable progress in implementing the community care reforms and working more closely together, the inspection revealed a lack of awareness of each other's roles and responsibilities, tensions around the efficiency of bed use and the pace of assessment, care planning and discharge and conflicts arising from increased and more complex workloads. Screening and referral systems were also very weak and effective monitoring was difficult.

Three years later, a more positive picture was to emerge (although still with some major reservations) from a similar study of hospital discharge arrangements in eight local authorities (Horne, 1998). Although things were *getting better*, there was still scope for further progress and a number of key issues remained:

- The difficulties of joint working are exacerbated by a lack of shared boundaries. This means that many health and social services workers are having to operate according to different eligibility criteria, assessment systems and service options depending on the geographical boundaries of the agency with whom they are collaborating.
- Factors which aid joint working include the support of chief officers, a willingness to cooperate among senior managers, an understanding of each other's perspectives and priorities, flexibility and common sense from frontline staff and jointly agreed mechanisms for monitoring information, measuring performance and resolving disputes.
- Identifying the best time to refer patients to social services could be difficult, although this could be aided by clear guidance and personal contact between health and social care staff.

- Levels of coordination with regard to assessment varied from area to area and contributions from community health and social care workers were seldom sought.
- The review of care plans was an acknowledged weakness.
- Disputes over strategic agreements could be overshadowed by a history of mistrust and mutual recrimination. While some social services managers considered the NHS continuing care criteria to be too stringent, some health managers felt that social services were not fulfilling their duty to provide community care. The resolution of such disputes could be aided by clarity of purpose, frequent meetings, multi-agency membership, avoidance of questioning multidisciplinary decisions, openness, clear and consistent procedures and documentation and the opportunity for decisions taken by joint panels to act as 'case law', refining policy and guidance for staff.

More recently, a number of further studies have served to increase our understanding of hospital discharge. For example:

- Adams (2001) emphasises the crucial role that can be played by housing services and by the voluntary sector in facilitating swift and effective hospital discharges.
- Research conducted by Carers UK suggests that carers are insufficiently involved in decisions about discharge from hospital and that their needs are not always taken into consideration when planning follow-up services in the community (Hill and Macgregor, 2001; Holzhausen, 2001).
- The causes of delayed hospital discharges are increasingly recognised to be many and varied, ranging from internal hospital delays to funding and service shortfalls within social care, and from housing-related reasons to choices made by service users and carers (see, for example, National Audit Office, 2000, 2003; Glasby, 2003a).
- While the problematic nature of hospital discharge is often associated with older people, it is equally an issue for other user groups, including people with mental health problems, learning difficulties or physical impairments (see Glasby, 2003a, for an overview).

However, perhaps the most crucial contribution to date has been made by a House of Commons Health Committee (2002) investigation into delayed hospital discharges. According to the Committee, around 7,000 people were delayed in hospital discharge in the second quarter of 2001-02 (occupying 6% of all acute beds), with delayed discharges costing the NHS around £720 million per year. In response to this situation, the Committee called for a number of key changes, including:

- Action to prevent unnecessary hospital admissions.
- A named person to coordinate all stages of the patient journey through hospital, up to and beyond discharge. This could take the form of a multidisciplinary

discharge liaison team, with a leader jointly appointed by the NHS and the social services department.

- A range of practical measures to reduce delays caused by internal hospital issues. Key issues include the need for earlier planning, the timing of consultant ward rounds, take-home medication, transport, discharge lounges and discharge coordinators.
- New government guidance on hospital discharge.
- A reconfiguration of services to avoid inappropriate admissions and facilitate timely discharges.
- Interim care arrangements to be made for patients waiting to enter a care home of their choice.
- A greater emphasis on supported housing and on the provision of aids and adaptations.
- The development of new technology (such as telemonitoring and telemedicine).
- Whole systems approaches to hospital discharge.

Above all, however, the committee was adamant that current difficulties associated with delayed hospital discharge could not be resolved without the creation of a single, integrated health and social care service (House of Commons Health Committee, 2002, p 58):

> The evidence we have heard simply strengthens our view ..., that the problems of collaboration between health and social services will not be properly resolved until there is an integrated health and social care system, whether this is in the NHS, within local government or within some new separate organisation. We recognise that [recent government initiatives] all add to the incentives for health and local authorities to work together, but they fall short of unifying the two agencies.... For many years there has been insistent exhortation for these bodies to work together. Unless there is a rapid change and clear evidence that the challenges of delayed discharges are being effectively managed by joint working, it will be further proof that leads to the inescapable conclusion that radical structural reform is required.

Building on the work of the Health Committee, a final contribution has been made by Glasby et al (2003), whose review of the literature on delayed hospital discharges and older people identifies a series of methodological limitations in the delayed discharge literature and raises a number of key questions about current policy and practice:

- Delayed discharge is the result of a wide range of factors and is a whole systems problem. For example, although attention often focuses on social services departments' handling of delayed discharge, internal hospital delays (such as waiting for take-home medication, delays in transport and the timing of consultant ward rounds) contribute to a significant number of delayed hospital discharges. Other factors include delays in community health services, delays in housing services and delays resulting from the choices made by service users and carers.

- The causes of delayed discharges differ from area to area, and agencies need to understand their own local solutions.
- Much of the existing research fails to consider the needs of older people with mental health problems or older people from minority ethnic communities.
- Delayed discharge is not the only issue: also significant are issues such as premature discharge, admission avoidance, the risk of inappropriate placements and delays in accessing community services.

Overall, the literature review raises a number of key issues about current policy and practice. In particular:

- Given the methodological limitations of the literature reviewed in this study, how evidence-based is current policy and practice?
- Given the complex and diverse nature of delayed discharges, is a measure like reimbursement going to be an adequate response? If delayed discharge is a whole systems problem, does reimbursement run the risk of damaging local relationships between health and social care?

In spite of all the policy initiatives, guidance and legislation described earlier in Chapter Three of this book, therefore, recent research findings indicate some improvement, but also a series of underlying and ongoing issues which have not yet been resolved. It is some of these unresolved issues which are illustrated below in the account of Andrew's experience of hospital discharge (see also Chapter Eight for further discussion of older people like Andrew with mental health problems).

Andrew's story

Andrew (87) is an Irish man living in an inner-city area. As his health began to deteriorate, he contacted social services and was assessed as needing home care three times a week to assist with shopping, bathing, housework, laundry and benefit collection. For several years, this care package proved sufficient to meet Andrew's needs and to help him retain his independence. As he grew older, however, his mobility began to decrease and his memory started to deteriorate. Worried that Andrew was becoming increasingly isolated and confused, Andrew's daughter, Mavis, contacted social services to request a reassessment of her father's needs. When the allocated social worker tried to telephone Andrew to arrange a home visit, however, she discovered from Mavis that Andrew had been admitted to hospital with severe chest pains. She therefore contacted the hospital with a view to visiting Andrew to assess his needs and discuss discharge arrangements with ward staff.

In the event, Andrew's discharge from hospital proved very different from that envisaged in the guidance outlined in Chapter Three of this book. First, ward staff failed to notify social services that Andrew had been admitted to hospital and might require additional support after discharge. To some extent this was understandable, since the cause of Andrew's chest pains had not yet been identified and it was not clear what was wrong with him or how long he would need to stay in hospital. When his social worker found out about Andrew's admission to hospital from his daughter, however, she felt that she should have been given greater notice that a new care package might well be required when the time came for Andrew to go home. Once again, this was not unreasonable, since her workload was such that she had to reprioritise her other cases in order to make time to see Andrew.

After this initial difference of opinion, a second point of tension soon arose. When Andrew's pains subsided his social worker was contacted and told that he had to be discharged that day. When the social worker reminded ward staff of a locally agreed 12-day timescale for assessment, they accused her of unnecessarily 'blocking' a hospital bed that could otherwise be used by people who needed it more than Andrew. As tempers rose, the social worker said that she had a heavy caseload, did not have the time to assess Andrew immediately and would comply with the agreed 12-day limit. In response, the ward sister told her that Andrew did not need to be in hospital and that she was "a typical social worker" unconcerned about pressures on the health service.

When the social worker completed her assessment, she was not satisfied that Andrew was capable of returning home. In her opinion, his mobility had decreased significantly and he was suffering from some form of cognitive impairment which might well be the onset of dementia. As a result, she requested that the ward refer Andrew to an occupational therapist (OT) before discharge could be considered. Despite assurances that her request would be carried out, no referral was made to an OT and the social worker decided to contact the department herself. This took place late on Friday afternoon after social services had closed for the weekend, with discharge planned for the following Monday. Concerned also about Andrew's reported bouts of confusion, the social worker sought to discuss the matter with ward staff, only to be told that this was a surgical ward which dealt with surgical issues and did not involve themselves in issues such as confusion. She therefore contacted a community psychiatric nurse (CPN) herself to request an assessment of Andrew's psychiatric condition.

By the time Andrew was discharged on Monday, therefore, the social worker and hospital staff were in complete disagreement about what had happened. As far as the hospital staff were concerned, they had allocated expensive and scarce resources in order to monitor an older man with chest pains until these pains subsided. They then sought to discharge him from hospital so that another patient could be admitted. From the social worker's perspective, however, ward staff had failed to refer a frail and confused patient to social services, an OT or a CPN, concentrating solely on his chest pains and neglecting his potential need for ongoing health or social support after discharge. In response, she wrote a letter of complaint to the hospital authorities, seeking to ensure that a similar situation could not happen again for other patients. The experience left workers in both agencies angry, frustrated and less willing to cooperate with colleagues from the other's discipline in the future.

Since his discharge, Andrew has returned to his home in the community, where his memory has continued to deteriorate. His chest pains have not returned and have never been explained, but he is now becoming noticeably more forgetful. This upsets him considerably, and he is frequently very tearful when he realises that he cannot remember where he put his keys or his wallet or the letter he was reading. It also distresses his daughter, Mavis, whom Andrew sometimes accuses of stealing his things when he cannot find them. Although he forgets a lot of what happens on a day-to-day basis, Andrew still remembers his time in hospital and says that it was a very negative experience. He was ill and in pain, yet felt that he must be being a nuisance because of the angry way in which the nurses and his social worker responded to each other. He recalls how he lay in bed listening to them argue about 'what to do with him', each accusing the other of not doing their job properly. He does not understand why this happened, but never wants to go through the ordeal of hospital discharge again. According to Andrew:

> "Waiting to go home was awful. Everyone was very nice to me, but they couldn't agree between themselves what should happen.... It didn't really seem to be anyone's fault – they were all kind people trying their best – but it just didn't work. No matter how hard they tried, they just couldn't find a way forward, and I was left stuck in the middle when all I wanted to do was to go home. I don't know what the matter is, but something needs to change so that other people don't have to go through what I did."

Exercise G: Andrew's story

1. What is your opinion of this hospital discharge?
2. How would Andrew and Mavis have felt during this process?
3. What could have been done differently to achieve a better hospital discharge?
4. From your knowledge of local health and social services and from the policy overview in Chapter Three of this book, what new partnership initiatives could have helped to provide more appropriate support for Andrew and Mavis?

For example:

- *Would a single assessment process help services adopt a more holistic approach to Andrew's and Mavis' needs?*
- *Will the development of intermediate care (see also Chapter Five) improve the experience of older people like Andrew?*
- *Would an integrated discharge team funded by a pooled budget help to provide more effective services?*
- *What impact will reimbursement have? Will it ensure that agencies communicate more effectively and plan for discharge, or will it make partnership working between health and social care more difficult?*
- *While a Care Trust might provide more coordinated support for Andrew, what else needs to be done to improve collaboration between hospitals and the community?*
- *Which other policies from Chapter Three could help to improve Andrew's experiences in the future?*

Good practice guide

- Always remember that the *focus should be on the needs of the service user* – in this case, Andrew's needs were almost forgotten amid debates about 'bed blocking' and the respective responsibilities of each agency.
- *Recognise the pressures that other workers face.* In this case study, ward staff felt under pressure to discharge Andrew as quickly as possible, while the social worker had a heavy caseload and simply could not cancel her other appointments to assess Andrew straight away. From the respective perspectives of the agencies and workers involved, both these stances were entirely legitimate.
- Remember that *the way you work* with other professionals will not only affect the service users involved, but *will also influence future attempts to engage in joint working.* In Andrew's case, the nurse had formed an opinion about the social workers she had met as not being concerned with pressures on the health service, and this made reaching a compromise and a way forward all the more difficult. Furthermore, both workers parted on bad terms, with joint working even less likely in the future as a result of the negative impressions formed during Andrew's discharge.
- *Regular personal contact* can be an aid to effective joint working. At a practice level, workers often find interagency collaboration easier when they already know the other practitioners involved and have good working relationships. This is particularly the case in hospitals, where joint working can be facilitated by the presence of social work teams in the hospital itself, with specific workers sometimes allocated to particular wards. In Andrew's case, the social worker was from an area team and did not know the health staff with whom she was trying to work. When difficulties arose, workers

who were better acquainted might have been able to achieve an informal solution. Here, the social worker felt she had no option but to make a formal complaint. Once again, this can create an atmosphere of mistrust which will make both parties less willing to engage in joint working in the future.

- Try to find *creative solutions* to joint problems rather than blaming each other. Here, the nurse and social worker sought to force each other to give way rather than trying to find a genuine solution to a difficult problem.
- *Do not allow yourself to become blinkered.* Rather than considering alternative service responses that might be able to meet Andrew's needs (rehabilitation, a transfer to a non-surgical ward, and so on), the social worker and the nurse continued to argue about whether Andrew should stay in hospital or be discharged home. Neither stopped to think of other ways of responding to Andrew's needs.
- Try to be *flexible* in your approach. When discussing Andrew's discharge neither worker was prepared to give ground, with one insisting that Andrew should be discharged that day and the other continuing to quote the 12 days allowed in local policy documents. Such intransigence benefited no one (least of all Andrew, who was traumatised by the experience of having workers argue over him).
- Try to take a *holistic view* of the service user's needs. In Andrew's case, the hospital adopted a very narrow, service-focused approach, monitoring his chest pains but neglecting other important issues as being outside its remit. People do not live their lives according to the categories laid down by service boundaries, and a degree of flexibility coupled with an ability to stand back and take an overview will be required if users' needs really are to be met in full.
- Always *carry out promises* made to a worker from a different discipline or agency. Here, the situation was exacerbated by ward staff agreeing to refer Andrew to an OT, but neglecting to do so. This could have been for a whole host of understandable reasons (the nurse may have forgotten due to a heavy workload, the OT may not have been available, ward staff could have had a handover and the need to make the referral might have been overlooked as the old staff went home and new staff started their shifts), but was interpreted by the social worker as being deliberately deceptive. This caused the situation to escalate unnecessarily.
- *Do not arrange discharges or agree discharge dates late on a Friday afternoon* when area social services teams will have closed for the weekend and cannot respond.
- Managers should ensure that *jointly agreed policy documents are accepted and implemented* at ground level. In Andrew's case, there was a local policy in place, but the nurse involved either did not know of it or did not agree with some of its contents. In her opinion, the issue at stake was the

'blocking' of a hospital bed, irrespective of any official agreements. To ensure joint acceptance, ownership and implementation of policies, joint training and joint monitoring may be a step forward.

Further reading

For those wishing to explore the complexities associated with hospital discharge in more detail, there are four main sources:

- The House of Commons Health Committee's (2002) inquiry into delayed discharges provides a comprehensive and critical overview, offering a series of recommendations for future policy and practice.

- Glasby's (2003a) *Hospital discharge: Integrating health and social care* is the first introductory textbook on hospital discharge, summarising our existing knowledge of the difficulties associated with hospital discharge, reviewing and critiquing government policy and offering a new framework for the way forward. Additional material is also available in Glasby (2002a, 2002b, 2002c, 2003c) and Glasby et al (2003).

- The Tertiary Care section of the Department of Health's website (www.dh.gov.uk/PolicyAndGuidance/OrganisationPolicy/TertiaryCare) contains further information on government policy with regard to hospital discharge and reimbursement.

- Melanie Henwood is a leading policy analyst with regard to hospital discharge, and a number of her works are cited in the Bibliography.

FIVE

Bert and Babu's story: rehabilitation and intermediate care

In many ways, the issues described in the previous chapter also have a direct bearing on the provision of rehabilitation services. As has already been suggested, attempts to achieve greater collaboration between health and social services with regard to hospital discharge have been hindered by two competing notions of good practice. On the health side there is a strong management concern "which is narrowly concerned with the cost-effective use of hospital resources (and hence with rapid through-put)", while on the social services side there is a commitment to "needs-led assessment and to choice for individuals" (Henwood and Wistow, 1993, p 6). In the same way that this creates tensions when it comes to discharging patients from hospital, it also makes the provision of effective rehabilitation extremely difficult, reducing opportunities for patients to undergo a period of convalescence and forcing them to make hasty (and often premature) decisions about their long-term care needs.

More recently, of course, traditional notions of rehabilitation have tended to be incorporated into the concept of intermediate care (services designed to prevent unnecessary hospital admissions, facilitate swift hospital discharges and prevent premature admission to permanent residential or nursing care). As a result, this chapter focuses on both rehabilitation and intermediate care, including two case studies to illustrate some of the issues facing older service users in this emerging area of policy and practice.

Exercise H: Rehabilitation and intermediate care

1. It is often said that health and social care services do not do enough to prevent older people being admitted to hospital, to support them in the community after discharge or to prevent them being admitted prematurely to residential or nursing care. What services are available in your area to cater for these needs?

2. It is also said that we have a very negative image of older people and tend to 'write them off' prematurely (that is, to assume that old age is a period of inevitable decline and admit older people directly to residential/nursing care when they may not need the services provided there). Do services in your area 'write older people off' and what could you do to help older service users maximise their potential?

Research findings/service issues

In 1992, a rehabilitation project was established in Hereford General and County Hospitals to prevent unnecessary admissions to residential and nursing home care (Littlechild et al, 1995). With the support of local social and health service workers, the project appointed a care manager to work with people aged 65 or over who were on the point of discharge from hospital and who had been assessed as needing residential or nursing home care. Significantly, the care manager had a small budget (in addition to the normal budget for services available to older people) to provide facilities beyond those currently available and was able to employ the services of an occupational therapist (OT).

Of the 34 cases assessed during the first six months, 76% people were able to avoid the permanent entry into residential or nursing care predicted for them when they were referred to the project (Table 5.1). This success was achieved by a combination of methods, with some users returning home with additional support and others undergoing a period of interim care out of the home. In all cases, the emphasis was very much on rehabilitation and convalescence, thereby preventing those users who entered residential care for short periods deteriorating and becoming permanent residents. Techniques for retaining this focus on rehabilitation included frequent home visits with key workers and care plans orientated towards regaining practical living skills.

To demonstrate the possibilities that effective rehabilitation offers, the story of one of the participants in this study (Bert) is included later in this chapter as a case study and the subsequent good practice guide is based on the key findings to emerge from an evaluation of the project (Smallwood and Jeffes, nd; Littlechild et al, 1995).

In 1997, the Audit Commission published a report on services for older people entitled *The coming of age*. Based on two previous studies of continuing care and the commissioning of community care services, the report identified a "vicious circle" (Audit Commission, 1997, pp 50-1) in which pressure on expensive hospital beds and the high use of nursing and residential care makes it hard to free up resources for alternatives that might start to ease the situation. These would include services to reduce the need for hospital admission on the one hand and investment in rehabilitation and convalescent facilities on the other.

Table 5.1: Predicted and actual destinations

Destination	Number of people (as predicted on referral)	Number of people (actual destination)
Residential home	24	3
Nursing home	10	1
Home with support	0	26
Deceased	0	4
Total	34	34

Source: Littlechild et al (1995, p 41)

While community services are beginning to develop, however, rehabilitation is seen as "the missing factor" (Audit Commission, 1997, p 60) in the care of older people. To break this circle, the Audit Commission was adamant that joint working was essential (p 50):

> The NHS and social services departments are locked together in the vicious circle. Although action by each agency is essential, action by one alone will not be enough. Their interdependence needs to be recognised if proper progress is to be made.... For example, if hospitals invest in more beds or facilities for rehabilitation, this will relieve the pressure on social services for residential and nursing homes. Similarly, if social services invest in effective preventative services such as respite care and intensive support at home for short periods during a crisis, then hospitals could benefit from fewer emergency admissions.... Joint planning and commissioning are therefore essential to explore alternative services.

To illustrate this point further, the Audit Commission provided a comparison of the situation in different authorities (A and B). Authority A spends three times as much per head on older people than authority B but invests much less in rehabilitation, joint working or community services. As a result, it has a much greater admission rate to residential and nursing home care, many more delayed discharges from hospital and many more readmissions to hospital.

Also in 1997, a number of findings regarding rehabilitation emerged as part of the Nuffield Institute's hospital discharge sub-study (Henwood et al, 1997) (see Chapter Four). In several of the study locations, the unavailability of rehabilitation facilities and disputes about service boundaries were common. In one authority respondents were worried that the contribution of social services funding to a multidisciplinary hospital-at-home scheme represented an unwelcome shift in organisational boundaries and responsibilities. This was described as "a big mistake", since it "sets in train the view that if you move hospital care into the community, social services will pay for it" (Henwood et al, 1997, p 38). Elsewhere, the virtual absence of any NHS rehabilitation services was felt to lead to inappropriate and avoidable placements in nursing and residential homes:

> There are such pressures to get people out of hospital, and the effect is that we have continued to place people in residential homes, even if that is not the best option.... There should be health purchased rehabilitation.

> People are put in nursing homes instead of in rehabilitation ... we don't provide the time for people to get better anywhere else than nursing homes. We have had people in nursing homes, and we have put in physio and OT support, and the person has gone home. I

think the medics tend to write them off. (Henwood et al, 1997, pp 38-9)

As awareness of the importance of rehabilitation grew, the Audit Commission and the King's Fund published the findings of two reviews commissioned to investigate the provision and clinical effectiveness of rehabilitation services. The first of these, *Trends in rehabilitation policy* (Nocon and Baldwin, 1998), drew attention to the unavailability and inadequacy of existing provision in different parts of the country, in some community settings and for user groups such as older people. Despite increases in specialist rehabilitation staff, opportunities for rehabilitation have actually decreased over the past decade. Although the report identifies a number of factors hampering the development of effective rehabilitation services and a number of ways forward, a key issue has been the lack of interagency collaboration. In particular, rehabilitation has traditionally been seen as the sole preserve of the health services, and its potential benefits have been neglected by social care providers. This has been exacerbated by cost shunting and boundary disputes, with many health authorities and social services departments unable to agree their respective responsibilities for rehabilitation. Despite this, the authors are convinced of the mutual benefits to be gained from effective joint working, emphasising the centrality of rehabilitation services if the length of hospital stays and the number of unnecessary residential and nursing home places are to be reduced. This will also be beneficial to users, who will receive a more efficient, coordinated service (Nocon and Baldwin, 1998, p 18):

> If users' needs are to be appropriately met, however, rehabilitation should be a comprehensive and integrated service which bridges gaps between different agencies. This will require a recognition that both health and social care agencies have an interest in improved rehabilitation outcomes. Funding will be needed to ensure that these services are provided, either by individual agencies or jointly. At a practice level, staff need to be aware of service users' potential needs for rehabilitation. They also need to recognise that the skills of other professional staff, including in those other agencies, can help to achieve rehabilitation goals.

The second Audit Commission/King's Fund review, *Effective practice in rehabilitation* (Sinclair and Dickinson, 1998), summarised the findings of some 56 systematic studies of the outcomes of rehabilitation, covering a range of disabilities, health problems, diseases and client groups. While much of the current research had significant limitations, many reviews presented positive findings, providing evidence of the clinical effectiveness of a range of rehabilitative interventions in a variety of conditions. Although little is known about the role of social care in isolation or as part of a coordinated package of care, the authors recognise the importance of providing rehabilitation services for older people, improving access for users and organising care in complex cases where multiple inputs are required from different disciplines and agencies. Above all, the review called for "a new clear focus on rehabilitation" as part of an attempt to "galvanise the present forces for change, provoke a more coherent research effort and stimulate real improvements in service delivery" (Nocon and Baldwin, 1998, p 28).

Despite the clinical effectiveness of rehabilitation emphasised by the Audit Commission and the King's Fund, however, a study conducted by the Social Services Inspectorate (SSI) has since pointed to the ongoing deficiencies in current provision (Horne, 1998). Of the eight authorities investigated, many had inadequate rehabilitation services (Horne, 1998, p 41):

> In about half the settings inspected the ability of the authorities to provide a choice of discharge options was significantly constrained by the limited rehabilitative services available. The respective positions taken by agencies on rehabilitation could be contentious and have consequences for individual patients, the professionals involved and the range of services available. At the agency level this served to obscure the expected roles of the parties, while at the patient level it confused the timing of an individual's assessment and the identification of the resources needed for their discharge.

Often, poor rehabilitative provision was associated, for social services departments at least, with an overreliance on expensive residential or nursing care, underdeveloped home care services, limited OT services and delays with adaptations or rehousing. Elsewhere, however, attempts were being made to develop imaginative, cost-effective and collaborative rehabilitation services, with one authority planning to turn two of its residential homes into specialist units providing intensive residential interagency input. These units would then act as a halfway house so that people could leave hospital to a safe rehabilitative environment in order to prepare themselves for returning home. While progress is being made, therefore, much remains to be done if effective rehabilitation facilities are to become established as part of mainstream service provision.

In the late 20th and early 21st century, policy documents and research which have previously focused on rehabilitation have begun to turn their attention to the concept of intermediate care. As noted in Chapter Three, intermediate care is designed to prevent unnecessary hospital admissions, facilitate swift and timely hospital discharges and prevent premature admissions to permanent residential and nursing care. According to circular 2001/001, intermediate care should be regarded as describing services that meet *all* the following criteria (DoH, 2001e, p 6):

- They are targeted at people who would otherwise face unnecessarily prolonged hospital stays or inappropriate admission to acute inpatient care, long-term residential care, or continuing NHS inpatient care.

- They are provided on the basis of a comprehensive assessment, resulting in a structured individual care plan that involves active therapy, treatment or opportunity for recovery.
- They have a planned outcome of maximising independence and typically enabling patients/users to resume living at home.
- They are time-limited, normally no longer than six weeks and frequently as little as one to two weeks or less.
- They involve cross-professional working, with a single assessment framework, single professional records and shared protocols.

To date, our knowledge of the effectiveness of intermediate care is limited by the relatively paucity of the evidence available. However, this is quickly beginning to change as more and more intermediate care services are being established and evaluated, and a number of preliminary findings are beginning to emerge. In particular, there are two key sources of information. The first is provided by the King's Fund (2002), whose intermediate care programme has led to the publication of a series of documents about intermediate care services. These cover topics such as:

- the role of intermediate care coordinators;
- mapping local rehabilitation and intermediate care services;
- financial issues;
- evaluating intermediate care.

However, particularly relevant to this summary of our existing knowledge is Vaughan and Lathlean's (1999) *Intermediate care: Models in practice*. In addition to describing a series of intermediate care projects in different areas of the country and based on different approaches to intermediate care, this overview summarises a number of key short- and long-term issues for debate (Box 5.1).

The second key source of information is the Department of Health's (2002c) *Intermediate care: Moving forward*. In addition to summarising our existing knowledge about intermediate care, this review of progress contains details of the available literature, current intermediate care evaluations and a number of forthcoming studies. In particular, the document identifies four key guiding principles for the development of intermediate care (and of services for older people in general):

1. *Person-centred care* (a commitment to ensuring that the needs and priorities of service users are placed at the heart of intermediate care).
2. *Whole systems working* (services that cut across traditional professional and organisational boundaries to provide a coordinated and holistic response).
3. *Timely access to specialist care* (intermediate care is about providing appropriate care for people in the right place and at the right time, and should never be seen as a mechanism for denying older people access to specialist care).

Box 5.1: Intermediate care: short- and long-term issues

Practical issues in implementing intermediate care:
- The need to allow sufficient time for planning and preparation: this is crucial if a strategic, whole systems approach is going to be achieved, but difficult if the scheme is financed by short-term funding. Time is also required for a service to become established and to begin to have an impact on mainstream health and social care services.
- Recruitment and retention of staff can be problematic.
- There is a need to ensure that innovations can be sustained and rolled out. Often, new services are supported by short-term funding and/or driven forward by a key individual. They are then fragile when the money runs out or the key individual moves on. Achieving equity of access to intermediate care across different geographical patches can also be difficult.
- Evaluation is crucial, but difficult to carry out effectively.
- It is important to consider the impact of new services on existing workloads.
- Intermediate care involves a shift in responsibility for patients' care from hospital to home. It is important, therefore, that issues of medical cover and of communication between different groups of workers are considered at an early stage.
- New partnership initiatives have the potential to enable workers to learn from each other and increase their own knowledge and skills. However, resistance to change and concerns about maintaining appropriate professional identities can hinder this.
- With new services, demand can increase over time.

Culture and context:
- How can we begin to change traditional ways of working and traditional patterns of service delivery?
- How can we begin to change public attitudes and expectations so that they learn to use and accept new services?
- How can we promote greater understanding of the different cultures and philosophies that exist in different sectors of the health and social care system?
- How can we improve the training of new workers so that they are able to work effectively together?
- How can we develop a whole systems approach at a time of rapid organisational change in health and social care?
- To what extent should we seek to reduce services elsewhere in order to redirect our efforts into new services like intermediate care? (Vaughan and Lathlean, 1999).

4. *Promoting health and active life* (intermediate care is about helping people to regain independence and fulfil their potential).

Next, *Moving forward* identifies a number of key success factors that may contribute to successful intermediate care services, before turning attention to four key issues which will need further consideration in the future. First, the document emphasises the importance of *addressing the needs of older people with mental health problems*. Amid concerns that some older people with mental health problems are being deliberately excluded from intermediate care in some areas, the government is clear that there is a need to ensure that services are responsive to the needs of this user group (see Chapter Eight of this book for further discussion). Second, the NHS system of *clinical governance* should be an essential feature of intermediate care so that quality of care and clinical safety can be demonstrated. Third, older people should have *timely access to medical assessment* so that their medical needs can be met. Finally, *housing services* have a crucial role to play in enabling older people to remain living independently in the community, and need to be a part of a whole systems approach.

In addition to the overviews provided by the King's Fund and the Department of Health, a case study from an intermediate care business plan provides a more detailed insight into some of the difficulties which can arise when trying to design and implement a new intermediate care service. While this has been described in more detail elsewhere (Glasby, 2003a, 2003b), the business plan revealed a number of difficulties that frontline agencies may face in trying to deliver the government's intermediate care agenda (Box 5.2).

A final insight into new intermediate care services comes from the House of Commons Health Committee (2002, pp 27-32), which is supportive of the concept of intermediate care, but concerned about a number of emerging issues:

- a lack of clarity about what the term 'intermediate' care means;
- the difficulty of achieving a strategic and integrated care system;
- a tendency to focus on providing 'more beds' rather than on reconfiguring existing services to invest more heavily in community services;
- inappropriate placements in some intermediate care schemes;
- fears that additional government money had been 'siphoned off' for other purposes;
- a lack of commitment to working in partnership with the independent sector;
- a tendency to 're-badge' existing services as intermediate care rather than develop new initiatives;
- the emphasis of government guidance on a six-week timescale rather than on working at the pace of the individual older person.

Overall, our own belief is that intermediate care is a concept with the potential to make a significant contribution to services for older people, but that further work may still be required to operationalise, evaluate and improve services to

Box 5.2: Practical difficulties in establishing intermediate care: a case study

- *Different professional values held by key stakeholders:* in drawing up a multi-agency business plan, different professionals and agencies had different attitudes towards a range of issues, including the balance between professional power and user choice, and between security and calculated risk taking by service users.
- *Different organisational agendas:* whereas several GPs were concerned that the proposed intermediate care facility was located close to their surgeries, the local hospital wished the service to be based in one of its own under-utilised buildings. In contrast, the social services department wanted to run the service from a former residential home and to be selected as the chosen provider.
- *The lack of shared boundaries between partner agencies:* drawing up the business plan involved contributions from primary care, secondary care, social care, housing and the independent sector, many of whom covered different geographical areas. As a result, local partners had to work in partnership not only with each other, but also with primary care organisations, social services departments and hospitals outside the local area.
- *The need to overcome significant organisational upheavals within individual partner agencies:* the business plan was compiled at a time when local primary care groups (PCGs) were in the process of becoming primary care trusts (PCTs), a local hospital was merging with a nearby hospital and the social services department was being reorganised.
- *Financial confusion:* some local health and social care agencies may be uncertain where the 'new' money pledged by central government has gone, how much money has been received and how much is actually available. In some areas, it is possible that the 'new' money may not be specifically set aside for intermediate care, but simply incorporated into the annual budget or used to compensate for shortfalls elsewhere in the system. In this particular case study, a significant proportion of the government's new money had already been spent in reducing previous overspends and taking account of inflation. With no additional money available, the business plan had to identify existing projects that could be incorporated into the proposed intermediate care facility, redirecting existing resources into the new service. Hardly surprisingly, this created significant tensions among local agencies and meant that the project was under considerable financial pressure before it had even begun.
- *The difficulty of establishing new services that span traditional boundaries within tight timescales* (Glasby, 2003a, 2003b).

ensure that they deliver on this potential in practice. That this is the case is illustrated later in this chapter by Babu, an older man whose experience of intermediate care enabled him to continue living in his family home, but which still had room for improvement.

Bert's story[1]

Bert is a 90-year-old widower who lives alone in a bungalow on the outskirts of a county town. He receives home care and visits a residential home for a meal and social activities once a week. On occasions he also has respite care at this home.

One winter, Bert was admitted to hospital with angina and chronic severe diarrhoea. He had severe leg ulcers and had recently fallen at home. A catheter had been fitted after Bert acquired a serious infection in hospital which exacerbated the diarrhoea. Hospital staff were of the opinion that Bert should be admitted to a nursing home because of his poor mobility and the need for catheter care. Bert had indicated a strong wish to return home, particularly as he missed his garden. As a result of this, the hospital arranged for a home visit to be carried out by the OT, but each time this was arranged the visit had to be cancelled because Bert became noticeably anxious and this, in turn, led to severe diarrhoea with incontinence. This pattern led to Bert becoming increasingly depressed and reinforced the hospital view that a nursing home was the most viable option.

Given this scenario the care manager hypothesised that Bert did want to return home but was frightened. He viewed the home assessment very much like a driving test – something to either be passed or failed. Because of the need to reduce 'bed blocking' in hospital, medical and nursing staff were unable to give him 'breathing space'. The care manager's solution was to engineer a placement that took the pressure off Bert, yet retained the goal of an eventual return home.

An interim stay in a nearby residential home for older people was arranged, therefore. This was a local authority home chosen by Bert. The officer-in-charge discussed the proposed admission with the named nurse, Bert and other ward staff. She felt that her establishment could cope with the catheter care required and the move subsequently went ahead. The district nurse, however, objected because she had not been consulted on the move and in retrospect it was acknowledged that this should have been discussed with her earlier.

On admission to the home the worst happened and Bert's condition deteriorated. His catheter became blocked and his incontinence increased. The home liaised with the GP who quickly became involved. The care manager hypothesised that the deterioration was related to the move and within a week the catheter was removed. The initial difficulties with the catheter and bowels were slowly overcome and Bert's self-confidence grew.

The home had appointed a key worker for Bert. In order to promote an effective attempt at rehabilitation, the care manager negotiated and paid for extra input from her to support a planned reintroduction to his home in conjunction with work from the OT. At first the OT simply visited Bert at the home. She then agreed a home visit with the key worker and Bert. In all she convened three such home visits and in the meantime the key worker continued to support and advise Bert at the home. She arranged a plan of visits to his bungalow which gradually increased the amount of time he spent there – sometimes with the key worker, sometimes alone.

Two care planning meetings took place at the local authority home. At the first meeting Bert asked for more time at the home and this was agreed to. In all he spent 12 weeks at the home, but is now back home and enjoying his garden.

Exercise 1: Bert's story

1. What is your opinion of this rehabilitation service?
2. How would Bert have felt during this process?
3. This was a time-limited pilot project. However, from your knowledge of local health and social services and from the policy overview in Chapter Three, what new partnership initiatives might be able to provide this sort of support for Bert?

Good practice guide

- Always try to be *flexible*. Here, the staff involved in Bert's care responded to developments and setbacks as they occurred, while still retaining sight of the original goal. This was crucial, for a failure to combine flexibility with an overall objective could have culminated in Bert returning home too early or in the entire attempt at rehabilitation being abandoned.
- Work at *the pace of the individual service user*, not of the service. In this case, Bert was given a 'breathing space' which enabled him to proceed at his own pace and rebuild his confidence before returning home.
- Consider the *feelings of colleagues* and be careful to acknowledge their skills and contributions. In Bert's case, time spent with the district nurse reassured her that nursing issues were not being overlooked and that planning was being done in a professional manner.
- Initial planning of innovative projects must ensure that everyone involved from all the agencies has a *common understanding* of the objectives and nature of the project and therefore *similar expectations* of what services can be provided. One of the ingredients of Bert's successful rehabilitation was the fact that workers from different disciplines were all committed to the same goal and were in agreement about how to proceed.
- The availability of *flexible, responsive interim resources* is critical. Here, Bert's recovery was aided by the fact that his care manager controlled a small budget and could use it flexibly to purchase care which was individually tailored to meet his needs.

> • Staff sometimes need to *'stand back'* and allow older people to do as much
>   as they can for themselves. Caring for people is often so instilled in some
>   workers that they find a more passive role uncomfortable. This has
>   implications for how people are trained. In this case, working with Bert in
>   an empowering way and allowing him to regain his independence in his
>   own time was crucial to the success of the rehabilitation programme.

Babu's story

Babu is a 82-year-old man who was born in Pakistan, but who emigrated to the
UK in the 1960s. Since the death of his wife some five years ago, he has been
living in a privately owned family house in an urban area with his daughter, her
husband and their four children. Although he is able to communicate with
others in English, this is not his first language and he finds it difficult to understand
technical terms or phrases which do not occur on an everyday basis. He also
speaks English with a very heavy accent and some white UK residents find it
difficult to understand him. He has arthritis and high blood pressure, and, as he
has grown older, his daughter has begun to support him with most aspects of his
personal care and prepares the food for all the family. Although registered with
a local GP, he does not receive any formal health or social services. However, he
does attend a voluntary lunch club for Asian older people that meets twice a
week in a local community centre.

  One day at the lunch club, Babu fell while trying to get into the minibus that
picks up and drops off members at the club. Although he did not seem to cause
himself significant injury, he was very shaken and bruised, and was temporarily
unable to bear his own weight. Although he initially refused to let the minibus
driver call an ambulance for him, Babu did allow his daughter to call the GP. On
visiting Babu, the GP felt that he required greater support than could be provided
at home in order to rest and recuperate from his accident, but that he did not
need the services provided in hospital. Babu was initially reluctant to receive
formal support, as the Asian community in his area had been campaigning for
some time to make local services more accessible to people from minority ethnic
communities. As well as distrusting formal service providers, Babu also wanted
to stay at home if at all possible and was keen for his daughter to care for him.

  In response, the GP was able to persuade Babu to try a local intermediate care
service based in a nearby nursing home. The scheme had recently been opened
by the mayor, and had been quoted in the local press (including the newsletter of
the local Pakistani community association) as an example of good practice.
Located in a private sector nursing home, the scheme offered 'step-up services'
to older people who are unable to remain at home but who do not need to go
to hospital. While support and personal care would be offered by care home
staff, additional input could be provided by OTs and physiotherapists from the
intermediate care team, who would assess Babu, help him to recuperate from his

injury and work with nursing home staff to design a rehabilitation programme. The service was free of charge and could last up to six weeks. While Babu was still reluctant to try this service, he was slightly reassured when his GP explained that the service would be able to meet his religious and cultural requirements. After discussing his options with his family, Babu agreed to go into the new step-up service.

Once at the nursing home, Babu made steady progress and was pleasantly surprised. The home itself was an attractive building with staff that were warm and friendly. In particular, Babu was made to feel as if the service he received was geared up to help get what he wanted (to go back home), and that nothing was too much trouble for staff in trying to achieve this aim. In addition, Babu's room was large, and the rehabilitation programme negotiated by the intermediate care team helped him to recover his mobility much more rapidly than he had expected. Although he had not mentioned this to anyone else, the fall had really damaged his confidence in his own ability to look after himself, and the intermediate care service gave him time and space to recover his confidence, his strength and his mobility in comfortable and friendly surroundings. Without this input, Babu now acknowledges that he would have been unable to cope at home and feels that he would have ended up in hospital. As it was, he felt well enough to return home after four weeks in the nursing home, and was able to go back to his home and to the lunch club with no further support from health and social services.

Unfortunately, however, some aspects of Babu's stay were not as satisfactory as he had been led to believe by his GP and by the publicity he had seen about the intermediate care scheme. Although located in a predominantly Asian area of the city, the home was staffed completely by white workers and Babu was the only older person from a minority ethnic community in the scheme. While vegetarian food was available, there was no access to halal meat and no separate facilities for Babu to pray. While staff made him feel very welcome, moreover, Babu began to feel that fellow residents did not like him. One older man in particular was very rude to Babu, saying that they "did not want his sort" there. Babu also found it difficult to communicate with fellow residents and with some members of staff, and was not offered access to an interpreter at any stage. Instead, he developed a close relationship with a member of staff who had recently done an evening class in Urdu–Hindi and was able to practise her new language skills by chatting to Babu. On one occasion, the issue of language caused significant debate, as a social worker attached to the intermediate care team seemed to feel very strongly that Babu should have access to a trained interpreter, while care home and therapy staff did not know how to access such services and said that they had no budget for such provision.

In addition, Babu felt that the care he received (while of high quality) could have been better coordinated. As far as he could tell, the daily living tasks he was supported to carry out and the exercises he had been asked to do were designed by the therapists from the intermediate care team, but tended to be put into practice by care home staff. At times, staffing difficulties within the home meant that Babu did not get the support he had been recommended as needing by the therapists and some of his exercises/daily living tasks had to be cancelled because there was no one available to help him with them. Babu also realised very early on that the intermediate care service was designed to help him do things for himself (to recover as much of his independence as possible). However, staffing shortages again prevented this from happening on some occasions, and some staff seemed to find it quicker and easier to do tasks for Babu rather than working with him to help him do them for himself. Although everyone was very supportive and welcoming throughout his stay, he feels that he could have gone home sooner had his intermediate care programme been more strictly implemented.

A final difficulty arose one evening when staff became concerned about the health of a fellow resident in the intermediate care project. Although they tried to call a GP out, the GP would not visit at night and said that the home should ring an ambulance. The home staff were not sure whether or not their concerns were serious enough to dial 999 and eventually decided to monitor the situation themselves. While the resident turned out not to need further medical treatment, Babu wondered what would have happened had the person's condition deteriorated and who would have been responsible for his medical care.

Overall, however, Babu feels that these limitations were a small price to pay for regaining his independence, and is quick to recommend the service to other older people at the lunch club.

Exercise J: Babu's story

1. What is your opinion of the service provided to Babu?
2. How would Babu have felt during this process?
3. What could have been done differently to improve the care offered to Babu?

Good practice guide

- *Never write older people off prematurely.* Here, Babu's story gives an example of the potential of intermediate care not only to reduce pressure on acute hospital services, but also to support older people to regain their independence and return to their chosen lifestyles. For Babu, the intermediate care service he received was sufficient to enable him to return home without any further input, and was highly valued by him. *Investing time* in someone early on, therefore, can bring a number of benefits later on and enable them to achieve their full potential.
- It is important to give older people the *time and space* they need to rebuild their confidence. In this case study, the intermediate care scheme provided the breathing space Babu needed to regain his independence.

- When working with older people at risk of hospital admission, adopting a *friendly and welcoming* approach can help the person feel at ease and begin to rebuild their confidence.
- Working in partnership can lead to the best of both worlds and the whole being *greater than the sum of its parts.* By combining a private sector nursing home with public sector therapists, the intermediate care scheme was based on a *public–private partnership* which seemed to be *drawing on the best of both partners* – the attractive building and committed staff of the nursing home and the rehabilitation skills of the intermediate care team. For some nursing homes, intermediate care represents a new and exciting way of working, and enables them to use spare capacity for a new type of service/patient. For some commentators, the care home sector may increasingly move towards this model of working in the future, and some homes are seeing intermediate care as 'the way to go'.

Despite obvious strengths, however, the scheme also had a number of limitations which illustrate some of the difficulties inherent in trying to establish an intermediate care service:

- Always ensure that intermediate care has appropriate *medical cover.* While Babu was unsure of the details, he was concerned about the apparent *lack of clarity* over who is supposed to provide *medical cover* for intermediate care. This is a significant problem at a national level (DoH, 2002c) and needs careful consideration when setting up a new service.
- Try to ensure that new partnerships are firmly *embedded in front-line practice.* Here, Babu's experience of intermediate care suggests that there were a number of problems coordinating the input of care staff (who spent the most time with service users and provided day-to-day support) and more specialist therapists (responsible for assessing Babu and designing his rehabilitation package). Unless all members of an intermediate care scheme are working together and pulling in the same direction, there is a risk that service users' care will be compromised and their rehabilitation hindered.
- Workers require sufficient *training* if they are being asked to behave in different ways (that is, working in a rehabilitative way rather than simply providing care). Here, some care staff seemed to be reverting to old ways of working when they were understaffed, doing things for Babu rather than with him.
- Although intermediate care has the potential to break the 'vicious circle' identified by the Audit Commission (1997), it is not a cheap option. Rather than cutting costs, intermediate care may actually increase them in the short term, providing intensive (and therefore expensive) inputs (with a view to improving outcomes and hopefully *saving money in the longer term*). In Babu's case, there does appear to have been a degree of understaffing in the nursing home, and this jeopardised his rehabilitation.

Above all, however, Babu's story illustrates the limitations of UK welfare services when trying to meet *the needs of people from minority ethnic communities*. Although based in a predominantly Asian area and publicising itself through a Pakistani community association newsletter, the scheme which supported Babu was not appropriate to meet his religious, language or cultural needs. While Babu felt welcomed and supported by individual staff members, he experienced direct and overt racism from fellow residents. Of particular concern is the failure to offer Babu access to an *interpreter* – a major oversight which might have meant that the assessment of his needs, the subsequent rehabilitation package and any consideration of follow-up needs in the community could be skewed or hindered by language barriers. Certainly, Babu cannot have had access to the same quality of care as people from a white UK background.

While it is crucial that intermediate care schemes (and all partnerships) take concerted action to ensure that their services are accessible to people from minority ethnic communities, different understandings of language and culture can also arise between workers from different professional backgrounds. Historically, social services departments have probably been more advanced than their healthcare colleagues in terms of considering and trying to respond to the needs of people from minority ethnic communities and have tended to provide/commission a larger range of translation/ interpretation services (see, for example, Dominelli, 1988; Thompson, 2001). In contrast, some NHS agencies have tended to resolve this issue by asking family members to interpret for them or relying on the language skills of frontline staff from the same ethnic background. Of course, neither of these latter approaches is acceptable. While the first compromises the confidentiality of the service user and puts the onus for communication onto the individual rather than onto the service, the second exploits frontline (and often low-paid) staff who are not necessarily trained in interpreting and who are not being employed for their language skills. In Babu's story, it is possible that these different approaches lay at the heart of what appeared to be growing tension between the social worker and other members of the intermediate care team about the importance of ethnicity and of people who do not speak English as a first language having access to trained interpreters.

Note

[1] Bert's story and the good practice guide which accompanies it are based on the rehabilitation project described at the start of this chapter and are taken from two accounts of the scheme, one unpublished and the other appearing in the journal *Elders* (see Smallwood and Jeffes, nd, and Littlechild et al, 1995). This project was established prior to the advent of intermediate care and was funded by the local social services department, but provides a practical illustration of the way in which services can be organised to enable older people to recuperate after hospital stays and achieve their desired lifestyles.

Further reading

A key contributor to the debate about the potential of rehabilitation and/or intermediate care services to make a positive difference to the lives of older people has been the Audit Commission, whose work is cited in detail in this chapter (Audit Commission, 1997; Nocon and Baldwin, 1998; Sinclair and Dickinson, 1998). Another key player has been the King's Fund (see, for example, Nocon and Baldwin, 1998; Sinclair and Dickinson, 1998; King's Fund, 2002).

For intermediate care, the Department of Health's (2002c) *Moving forward* document summarises the main challenges and issues as local services seek to develop their intermediate care provision. A more critical approach is offered by the House of Commons Health Committee (2002), which is supportive of the concept of intermediate care but concerned about the way in which services are developing on the ground.

For further information on intermediate care, visit the website of the national evaluation being undertaken by the Universities of Birmingham and Leicester (www.prw.le.ac.uk/intcare). Also useful is Petch's (2003) summary of what we currently know about older people's experiences of intermediate care.

SIX

Ben's story: continuing care

In addition to tensions during hospital discharge and a lack of rehabilitation facilities, the confusion surrounding the health and social care divide is particularly evident with regard to continuing care. For those with high-level needs requiring complex and ongoing support, the decision as to whether they are eligible for free NHS care (known as NHS continuing care) or means-tested social care is a major issue. Although government guidance has sought to encourage health authorities and social services departments to clarify their respective responsibilities in this area, the evidence both from research and from the experiences of older people such as Ben (see later in this chapter) suggests that a series of ongoing and underlying problems remain.

Exercise K: Continuing care

1. How might an older person with continuing healthcare needs be feeling about their current situation and about what the future may have in store for them?
2. How might their family be feeling?
3. Are there particular situations or services where the responsibilities of health and social care could overlap?
4. If so, what steps could practitioners and services take to ensure that the services offered to older people are as coordinated as possible?
5. Which of the policies in Chapter Three might help to achieve this goal?

Research findings and service issues

In 1992, a review of recent policy and research identified the continuing care of older people as "the Achilles' heal of the community care reforms" (Henwood, 1992, p 28). By extending local authority responsibilities for nursing home care, the NHS Community Care Act (NHSCCA) was in danger of creating a "hazy boundary and disputed no-man's land between health and social care", with patients too well for the former but too ill for the latter (Henwood, 1992, p 28). In support of this assertion, the review cited research findings which identified a considerable overlap between dependency levels in different types of care. These suggested that not only is there a discrete and identifiable group of people requiring NHS continuing care, but that this group is cared for in a range of settings, apparently irrespectively of their needs. Such a situation mirrors that described by Huws Jones (1952) in Chapter Three, exactly 40 years previously, pointing to an ongoing failure to promote effective joint working with regard to continuing care.

The following year, research carried out for the Social Services Inspectorate (SSI) highlighted the uncertainties surrounding the extent of NHS responsibility for continuing care (Henwood and Wistow, 1993). Of the six authorities studied, this issue remained more or less unresolved in every locality, with decisions about how to allocate care based on ad hoc, individual decisions rather than on agreed policies. In one authority, the distinction between those qualifying for NHS continuing care and those having to contribute to their own fees in a home funded by social services was based not on clinical differences, but on whether or not individual patients were actually prepared to pay for their care. Thus, those who remained as NHS patients often did so not necessarily because they needed to, but because they had refused to pay for alternative services. Everywhere, the issue was felt to be a 'grey area' in between the boundaries of health and social care, and one which could have significant implications:

> The widespread confusion which surrounded policy in this area was about far more than the delineation of service boundaries, and financial responsibilities between health and social services. Many respondents were extremely concerned about the implications for individual patients or service users. The question of where the financial and caring responsibilities of the NHS should end was, therefore, exercising many policy makers and practitioners within our six localities. The issue is also one which arises for client groups other than elderly people, and indeed applies to any people for whom the NHS has formerly had long stay responsibilities. Repeated legal challenges and judicial reviews were seen as likely to emerge in an attempt to clarify what remains a very uncertain, but profoundly important, issue. (Henwood and Wistow, 1993, p 36)

In 1995, a series of focus groups held in five English localities identified two further problems around continuing care (Henwood, 1995). The first concerned the impact on individual service users of the changing boundaries between health and social care. As social services took on greater responsibility for care traditionally provided by the NHS, users were having to pay for services which were previously free. As one voluntary sector worker explained:

> Many older people feel insulted about the means testing of services. They believe they have paid in all their lives and are now being cheated by changing rules. The result is a great deal of anger. People are afraid of the financial implications of asking for help. (quoted in Henwood, 1995, p 23)

A second issue was the difficulty of responding to people with complex long-term needs, especially those with both physical and mental health problems. Where the agencies involved could not agree an appropriate service for such people, the danger was that they would be placed in facilities which did not meet their needs at all.

Two years later, findings from a study of continuing care arrangements in six localities were published by the Community Care Division of the Nuffield Institute for Health (Henwood et al, 1997). In areas where there was a history of joint working (three of the six), the process of drawing up policies and eligibility criteria had been relatively straightforward; elsewhere progress was slow. Although all six localities had been able to produce joint policies, the degree of 'jointness' was often not apparent. In particular, there was little evidence of coherence and consistency between health and social services policies and criteria, very little emphasis on developing joint commissioning strategies and a suggestion that many social services had found themselves having to respond to a health authority agenda, often led by consultants. This could create tension between social services managers and frontline practitioners, with the latter feeling that their department had simply acquiesced with unacceptable health service demands. For managers, the failure to take a firm line tended to be justified in terms of the importance of maintaining good relations with the health authority. While it was still too early to judge the success of the continuing care agreements, most respondents reserved judgement until they could see how the policies and criteria worked in practice.

In 1998, further research by the SSI found evidence of ongoing problems with regard to continuing care (Horne, 1998). Despite the requirement that health and social services should have joint continuing care agreements, more than half of the eight authorities inspected had not achieved this. Although a series of policies had been put out for consultation, disagreements had arisen over issues such as the scale of health funding, the strictness of the eligibility criteria and the practicality of implementing the policy. This was particularly the case in areas with a history of mistrust between health and social services. Here, it was not uncommon for social services managers to feel that the continuing care criteria were too stringent and effectively precluded any possibility of the NHS funding services or agreeing to share funding with social services. Conversely, some health authority managers believed that social services were not fulfilling their obligations to provide community care. These relations were also exacerbated by the turnover in managerial staff and the pressures of the local government reorganisation which was taking place at the time.

In 1999 a study of continuing care criteria and policies in six health authorities highlighted the way in which patients' rights to publicly funded healthcare had been eroded by the introduction of eligibility criteria under the 1995 continuing care guidance (South, 1999). After analysing the requirements for fully funded NHS care, the study demonstrated how the criteria developed by the six health authorities focused on those who required specialist care and supervision with regard to particular clinical conditions. This meant that other patients with high-level but non-specialist health needs were being denied free healthcare and would be liable to pay for some or all of their care in a nursing home. The author of the study considered this to represent a formal loss of entitlements and a significant stage in the rationing of healthcare.

Also in 1999, the Royal College of Nursing (RCN) undertook a study of 25 randomly selected health authorities (approximately a quarter of all health authorities in England and Wales) (Dixon et al, 1999). This research was based on a legal analysis of continuing care policies in the light of the Court of Appeal judgement on the Coughlan case (see Chapter Three), focusing on the eligibility criteria which were used to assess whether a person was entitled to NHS funding in a nursing home. Overall, the study found that almost 90% of the health authorities were using criteria that "were either likely or highly likely to be unlawful" (Dixon et al, p 40) and might be vulnerable to a legal challenge in the light of the Coughlan judgement.

In addition, the study also highlighted the lack of consistency between different health authorities, with some authorities not accepting responsibility for *anyone* needing nursing home care. A small telephone survey of 10 expert nurses working with older people on the application of the eligibility criteria in practice found that assessments "are often time-intensive, influenced by funding needs and not multidisciplinary in approach" (Dixon et al, 1999, p 5). There was little evidence of the use of reliable assessment tools and there was little transparency or clarity in decision making. On the basis of the findings from this small study, the RCN report concluded that too much time and effort is focused on frustrating debates about the application of the eligibility criteria and which agency should take responsibility for funding and too little on determining and responding to the health needs of patients.

In 2000, Bridges et al published the findings of research, carried out in 1997 in one London health authority, which was designed to evaluate the implementation of local continuing healthcare policies. The study included 82 older people, 46 with physical impairments and 36 with mental health needs who had been placed in a range of settings in the first 10 months since the implementation of the new policy in April 1996. The aims of the study were to determine the characteristics of the older people in the sample who had been assessed as eligible for NHS-funded care, chart their progress since placement and examine the arrangements individual units had in place for their care. The data was collected via a questionnaire administered to a senior member of nursing staff who knew the older people in the units in which they were placed.

The authors of the report acknowledged that this was a small study in one authority and made no claims about its representativeness. However, some interesting themes emerged which require further investigation:

- Both groups of older people were highly dependent but a small number required rehabilitative care and a proportion were perceived by the nurses as having improved since their placement began. There was little clarity in the 1995 guidance about how rehabilitation integrates with continuing care.
- The needs of the older people in the study required a high level of nursing skill yet the guidance offered little direction about the type of medical cover and levels of qualifications required in such units.
- Most of the nursing care was offered by nurses within the units rather than other specialist nurses and it is not clear whether this is the kind of 'specialist nursing' referred to in the guidance.

However, in recent years, it seems that few of the issues identified in this chapter have been resolved. Despite the issuing of new continuing care guidance in 2001 (see Chapter Three of this book), controversy over funding for long-term care for older people remains a critical issue between health and social services. In February 2003, the Health Service Ombudsman published a report outlining the issues which had arisen from the 13 complaints that her office had received in the previous 18 months about NHS funding of long-term care. In particular, the Ombudsman identified five key issues which emerged from the complaints, most of which concerned events which took place before the issuing of the 2001 guidance:

- informing and involving patients and their relatives;
- developing eligibility criteria for NHS-funded care in line with guidance issued in 1995;
- reviewing eligibility criteria in the light of the Coughlan judgement (July 1999);
- the national framework for NHS-funded care;
- assessment against criteria.

Involvement and information

Patients' and relatives' complaints about involvement and information are all too familiar – not being sufficiently involved in decisions about moving into a care home and being given inadequate information about how decisions are made or what the financial implications are. Where the move is made from hospital there are complaints about pressure being put on patients to make decisions, views of patients and relatives not being taken into account and inadequate explanation of criteria and procedures. The Health Service Ombudsman highlighted difficulties in communication between those responsible for setting the eligibility criteria and those practitioners who carry out clinical assessments of patients' needs against the criteria.

Developing eligibility criteria in line with 1995 guidance

Eligibility criteria for NHS-funded continuing care following the 1995 guidance varied from one area to another as health authorities had to specify their own local criteria within the broad national framework. Some patients and their relatives have made complaints about variations in eligibility criteria and, while such differences in themselves may not indicate maladministration, the Health Ombudsman had seen some local criteria which "appeared to be significantly more restrictive than the guidance permitted" (Health Service Ombudsman, 2003, p 5).

Taking the Coughlan judgement into account

As outlined in Chapter Three, following the Coughlan case, health authorities were required to review and, where appropriate, revise their criteria in line with the judgement. Where changes were made, they were also required to reassess the eligibility of patients for NHS-funded care. The Health Service Ombudsman has found evidence of some health authorities making little effort to review their criteria and reassess patients and little encouragement or monitoring from the Department of Health for them to do so. Strategic health authorities now have the responsibilities of health authorities and PCTs now hold the relevant budget so the Health Service Ombudsman has recommended that these two bodies should:

• Review the criteria used by their predecessor bodies, and the way these criteria were applied, since 1996. They will need to take into account the Coughlan judgement, guidance issued by the Department of Health and the Ombudsman findings.
• Make efforts to remedy any consequent financial injustice to patients, where the criteria, or the way they were applied, were not clearly appropriate or fair. This will include attempting to identify any patients in their area who may wrongly have been made to pay for their care in a home and making appropriate recompense to them or their estates (Health Service Ombudsman, 2003, p 6).

The Ombudsman also recommended that the Department of Health takes a more proactive role in supporting and monitoring the work that the strategic health authorities and primary care trusts (PCTs) have to do in this area.

The national framework for NHS-funded care

As Chapter Three indicated, the Health Service Ombudsman has received complaints from patients and relatives about the lack of transparency and fairness in the criteria for NHS funding of long-term care. In her view, the 2001 guidance was weaker than the previous guidance and gave no clearer definition of when the NHS should fund long-term care, rather giving a list of factors to be taken into account. In view of this she has recommended that:

> The Department of Health should review the national guidance on eligibility for continuing NHS health care, making it much clearer in new guidance the situations when the NHS must provide funding and those where it is left to the discretion of NHS bodies nationally. This guidance may need to include detailed definitions of terms used and case examples of patterns of need likely to mean NHS funding should be provided. (Health Service Ombudsman, 2003, p 7)

Assessing against criteria

In looking at the ways in which health authorities have applied their local criteria to individual patients, the Health Service Ombudsman found a range of practices. Some authorities have produced detailed guidance on the criteria and how to apply them, ensuring some level of consistency within an area. In others there has been little or no advice for clinical staff on how to apply the procedures, resulting in lack of consistency and fairness. The Health Ombudsman concluded that the Department of Health has not been forthcoming with help on methods or tools of assessment and recommends that it should consider "how to link assessment of eligibility for continuing NHS health care into the single assessment process and whether it should provide further support to the development of reliable assessment methods" (Health Service Ombudsman, 2003, p 8).

Overall, the issue of NHS funding of long-term care remains a contentious one. For strategic health authorities and PCTs, the report from the Health Service Ombudsman has major resource implications if they must identify patients who have already been negatively affected by the application of over-restrictive criteria and make appropriate redress. For patients and their relatives, such decisions will have had significant financial effects if they have been incorrectly made to pay for their care in a home. Eligibility for free health-funded nursing care is one of the issues illustrated in the following case study.

Ben's story

Ben is a 85-year-old man living in a large urban area and was admitted to a general hospital after a stroke. Once in hospital, Ben made only a limited recovery and, after a long stay, it was clear that he would not be able to return to his own home. Ben had one son, Gerald, who visited daily and he made it clear to hospital staff that he would not be able to offer his father the kind of support he would need at home. Ben's mobility remained severely restricted, he had a peg-feed fitted for feeding (a tube into his stomach to enable him to take in food), a catheter fitted and some faecal incontinence. Ben's speech was impaired but, with patience, people who knew him well could understand him.

Ben's consultant said that Ben no longer required hospital care and arrangements should be made for his discharge. There were a number of health and social care professionals involved in planning Ben's transfer from hospital. In Ben's area, the social services department and the former health authority had agreed joint criteria for funding the care of people with community care and continuing healthcare needs as required by the government's 2001 guidance (see Chapter Three of this book). These criteria were readily accessible to users and carers in an easily readable format, were available in community languages for people from minority ethnic communities and were extremely explicit in explaining what sort of treatment and services patients could expect from each of the respective agencies. Using the criteria, patients' health needs were assessed and the patient placed into one of six categories, with levels 1, 2, 3 and 4 funded by social services, level 5 jointly funded by social services and health and level 6 funded by health alone.

The hospital social worker did an assessment and, in conjunction with the ward staff, assessed Ben's considerable physical needs as being most appropriately met by a nursing home. They assessed Ben's needs as fitting into their Level 4 category which meant that, as Ben owned his own house and lived alone, he would become a self-funding resident in a nursing home.

The social worker talked with Ben throughout the assessment process and arranged to meet Gerald when he was visiting. However, the social worker was taken aback at Gerald's reaction when she told him the outcome of the assessment. Gerald was conversant with the health and social services access criteria as he was in a dispute with the social services department regarding his mother-in-law. Until three years ago, she lived in a town covered by a neighbouring local authority and a nearby PCT. She had since moved into a nursing home with the

---

Continuing healthcare criteria

Level 1: person needs minimal help to remain at home (social services funded).

Level 2: person needs help with essential activities of daily living (social services funded).

Level 3: people with more complex needs who need help with the majority of their personal care (social services funded).

Level 4: people who are highly dependent and need nursing care or supervision (social services funded).

Level 5: people who need a higher level of care than would normally be provided in a nursing home or who have an anticipated life expectancy of less than 12 months (health and social services funded).

Level 6: people with complex/unstable healthcare needs, requiring nursing and/or medical care in hospital or in a specialist service (NHS funded).

onset of dementia and her house was sold to pay for her care. Her private funding had now run out and there was a dispute between the two social services departments as to who would fund her care. However, in addition, the social worker from the authority to which she had moved (who worked in the same office as Ben's social worker) was saying that his mother-in-law may be eligible for some funding from health as her needs were more specialist than could be provided for in the current nursing home. Gerald claimed, however, that his mother-in-law's condition initially deteriorated fast but that it had not changed for a year. Did that mean she would have been eligible for health funding a year ago? If so, was she eligible for a retrospective assessment as it had significant financial implications?

Gerald was a well-known figure in the local community and had already alerted his local councillor to the situation with his mother-in-law. When the social worker told him that his father would be entirely self-funding in a nursing home, he was able to quote two of the access criteria for Level 5 which he believed would make his father eligible for a combination of social services and health funding, of which the health proportion would be entirely free of charge:

- your physical or mental health is frequently changing and you need specialist medical help;
- your care is very difficult to manage because of your combination of mental and physical health problems.

The social worker decided that she needed multidisciplinary support and called in the discharge planning sister from the PCT who agreed to do an assessment within the next few days. By this time Gerald had begun to get a reputation among the ward staff and within the social services team as being argumentative, pushy and prepared to use his connections to get what he wanted on behalf of his father. The discharge planning sister carried out her assessment and, after discussing the case with some of the medics involved in Ben's care, agreed with the previous outcomes – that Ben came into the Level 4 access criteria:

- people who are highly dependent and need nursing care or supervision.

The discharge planning sister met with Gerald to discuss the outcome and found a very anxious but committed man who was determined to fight for what he thought his father deserved. Gerald insisted that, in his view, his father fell within the Level 5 criteria and asked whether there was anywhere to go with an appeal against the decision of the professionals. The discharge planner agreed to call a multidisciplinary case review so that all the professionals who had seen Ben could pool their information and come to a final decision.

Gerald agreed to attend but was resigned to the fact that if all the people involved so far had said his father fitted Level 4 criteria, then that was what the final decision would be and there was really no point of a further meeting. The discharge planning sister went ahead and arranged the meeting, ensuring that she fully involved Ben and Gerald in making it at a convenient time when Gerald would be visiting the hospital anyway. By the time the review took place, it was three weeks since the original assessment and Ben was identified by the hospital as a 'delayed transfer of care'. Ben did not himself attend the case review.

At the case review, the social worker and the discharge planning sister gave their assessments of Ben's needs. Gerald explained why he thought his father met the Level 5 criteria. Also at the review was Ben's consultant who had not previously offered an opinion on Ben's eligibility for continuing healthcare. He was of the view that Ben *did* fall within Level 5 as he fitted the criteria of:

• people who have an anticipated life expectancy of less than 12 months.

This was an unexpected contribution but the final outcome of the case review was that Ben should move to a nursing home, partly self-financed and partly funded by the PCT. The consultant's view of Ben's prognosis was not a surprise to Gerald, but he was rather taken aback to have heard it expressed for the first time and in such a stark manner within the case review setting. He did, however, have an overwhelming sense that justice had been done on behalf of his father and that he had got what he deserved in terms of financial support. More than anything, he was surprised that this was not a decision that was 'done and dusted' before the review as he had suspected and was impressed that an alternative outcome had been reached.

Ben moved into a nursing home three weeks later where he lived for two months before he died.

Exercise L: Ben's story

1. What is your opinion of this situation?
2. How would Ben and Gerald have felt during this process?
3. What could have been done differently to achieve a better outcome for Ben and Gerald?
4. From your knowledge of local health and social services and from the policy overview in Chapter Three, what new partnership initiatives could have helped to provide more appropriate support for Ben?

For example:

- *Would a single assessment process help services adopt a more holistic approach to Ben's needs?*
- *Could local services consider use of one of the Health Act flexibilities?*
- *What impact would an older person's Care Trust have on people in Ben's position?*
- *How would Ben's situation have differed if the government had implemented free personal care as recommended by the Royal Commission on Long Term Care?*
- *How confident are you that recent changes in continuing care guidance are likely to make a significant impact on older people like Ben given the longstanding nature of many of the issues at stake?*
- *Which other policies from Chapter Three could help to improve the experiences of people like Ben in the future?*

Good practice guide

- Ensure that *sensitive information* is not disclosed for the first time in case reviews. In this case, Gerald had been given no indication of his father's prognosis and it had not been discussed with Ben himself.
- Assessments are time-consuming for professionals and often exhausting for older people who feel they are being asked the same questions time and time again. *Multidisciplinary assessments* are important in bringing together the views of different people, but they need to be coordinated to make more efficient use of people's time and skills. In Ben's case, it was three weeks between the first assessment by ward staff and the multidisciplinary case review.
- Ensure that all members of the multidisciplinary team are *fully involved* in decisions. Here, the consultant did not seem to have been involved until a very late stage, and yet had a decisive contribution to make.
- If it is not possible to arrange a multidisciplinary case review where everyone meets together within a reasonable length of time, how else can the *views of the people involved* be gathered and a decision made? In this situation, it is unlikely that a review would have been held if Gerald had not insisted, but the outcome would have been very different without the consultant's opinion.
- Good multidisciplinary working involves *shared decision making* and not taking it personally when the outcome goes against your professional judgement. In this situation the discharge planning sister may have felt undermined by the consultant, but that was to do with the process by which the decision was made rather than the decision itself. Professionals must respect the views of others and be clear on what basis decisions are made.

- It is important that older people and their families have *full possession of information and clear explanations of how and why decisions have been made.* Here, Gerald was in full possession of the eligibility criteria which was easily accessible, detailed and explicit. Even so, the definition of 'a higher level of care than would normally be provided in a nursing home' was open to interpretation. In the end, Gerald's view of his father's eligibility for Level 5 was upheld, but on quite different criteria from his previous discussions with nursing and social work staff.

- In some cases, particularly where older people do not have relatives to speak up on their behalf, professionals may find themselves acting as an *advocate* as well as an employee of the agency. This can be a difficult role and one which may bring them into conflict with other professionals. Where possible it may be better to seek *independent advocacy* for the older person. If Ben had not had Gerald to represent him, it is likely that he would have been moved to a nursing home as a self-funding resident.

- Try *not to make assumptions* about older people or their families based on other people's experiences. Here, the discharge planning sister had been given a rather negative picture of Gerald, but instead she found someone who was well-informed, determined and desperate to ensure his father was treated fairly.

- How do your eligibility criteria and the interpretation of them compare with neighbouring areas? Are there any *cross-boundary*/regional discussions? In this situation, it is likely that at least two social services departments and two PCTs were going to be involved in a dispute over their responsibilities regarding Gerald's mother-in-law.

Further reading

Detailed findings of the study of continuing care policies in 25 health authorities in England and Wales, after the Coughlan judgement, can be found in Dixon et al (1999). The publication is out of print and can only be obtained from the Royal College of Nursing Library, 20 Cavendish Square, London WM1 OAB or by e-mail (lending.services@rcn.org.uk).

Current issues for debate are dealt with in detail in the Health Service Ombudsman's report (Health Service Ombudsman, 2003); also useful is Malin (2000).

SEVEN

Ivy's story: domiciliary care in the community

With reductions in the number of long-stay hospital beds and greater emphasis on the provision of both health and social care in more homely, non-institutional settings, the issue of domiciliary care has become increasingly prominent in recent years. As the nature of traditional service provision has changed, the dependency of service users receiving care in the community has increased, creating more complex caseloads for the workers involved and raising new demarcation disputes between community nurses and home carers in particular. This has been most clearly evidenced by the gradual transition of traditional home help schemes (providing practical assistance with tasks such as shopping and cleaning) into home care services (providing a significant amount of personal care previously considered the role of the health services). While debates about the health and social care divide with regard to community services have traditionally been less fierce than those surrounding institutional care, therefore, they have been no less significant (Means and Smith, 1998a).

Exercise M: Domiciliary care in the community

1. How might an older person who is beginning to lose their independence in the community be feeling about the possibility of contacting health/social services or about the future?
2. How might their family be feeling?
3. Are there particular situations or services where the responsibilities of health and social care could overlap?
4. If so, what steps could practitioners and services take to ensure that the services offered to older people are as coordinated as possible?
5. Which of the policies in Chapter Three might help to achieve this goal?
6. What do older people think about home care services and what do they value about this form of provision (after completing this exercise, compare your answers with Boxes 7.1 and 7.2 later in this chapter).

Research findings and service issues

Initially, research on domiciliary services published prior to the NHS Community Care Act (NHSCCA) tended to emphasise a lack of integration between carers employed by the health service and those employed by social services (see, for example, Bebbington and Charnley, 1990; Sinclair et al, 1990). In particular, disputes over responsibilities for areas of work such as personal care led to major role conflicts, creating gaps and overlaps in service provision. However, research undertaken during the community care reforms has highlighted the way in which the boundaries between health and social services have started to shift. Between 1992 and 1994, for example, a series of surveys was carried out in an inner-London health authority as part of a review of district nursing services (Barrett and Hudson, 1997). On the appointed study days, all district nurses from the area were asked to fill in forms detailing their clinical and non-clinical work, their time spent travelling and the number and characteristics of the patients they saw. Although the number of patients remained fairly stable over the three years, there was a marked increase in the number of very elderly patients (aged over 85) and the number living alone. Even more significant was a change in the pattern of care provided, with a much greater emphasis on technical nursing care and less on personal care in 1994 than in 1992. This had implications for skill mix, requiring more trained nurses and fewer nursing auxiliaries. The findings also led the researchers to wonder what had happened to the less dependent patients who would previously have been on the district nursing caseload, receiving personal rather than technical care. One hypothesis put forward by Barrett and Hudson (1997) is that these patients are now being seen by social services care assistants. This would seem to suggest that the boundaries between health and social care in the community are shifting in a manner similar to that already identified earlier with regard to institutional care.

In 1995, a Social Services Inspectorate (SSI) study of home care services in six local authorities found variable arrangements for liaison with health authorities (DoH/SSI, 1995b). While the respective responsibilities of each agency were generally clear at an operational level, there were still areas of difficulty arising from early discharges and disputes about responsibility for bathing services, the administration of medication and the supply of incontinence pads. One year later, a second report covering findings from a further nine authorities confirmed many of these issues, reiterating the need to focus attention on particular areas of friction between health and social care (DoH/SSI, 1996). These included responsibilities for personal care tasks, which was increasingly being undertaken by home carers, despite the fact that they had not always been trained to perform this role.

In 1998, the Nuffield Institute for Health published results from a study carried out with the United Kingdom Homecare Association (Henwood et al, 1998). This research aimed to investigate which aspects of the domiciliary care service were most important to service users and carers and to develop a framework to help commissioners and providers of care to develop appropriate services. The research was conducted over three sites and involved 46 service users (the majority of whom were over 70) and 12 carers. Rather than shedding light on the health–social care divide, the study suggested that older people value three different things about home care, irrespective of who it is provided by (see Box 7.1).

Box 7.1: Domiciliary care and older people's priorities

1. Organisation and management of the service:
- clarity over the type of care provided and how much flexibility there was over tasks;
- continuity of care – users appreciated that it was not possible to always have the same worker but resented unexplained and frequent changes;
- sufficient time for each client;
- clear communication about changes of arrangements;
- clear identification about who to contact about problems/complaints;
- regular reviews;
- review and supervision of standards of care.

2. Characteristics of care staff:
- mature;
- kind and understanding;
- professional;
- friendly;
- competent and adequately trained;
- reliable.

3. Contents of care:
- greater flexibility in what is provided;
- matching services to clients' needs;
- adapting services to meet changing needs. (Henwood et al, 1998)

Similar findings have also emerged from a more recent study conducted in Manchester which was designed to involve older service users in designing home care specifications (Raynes et al, 2001). The sample included people invited to participate from the Chinese and Asian communities in Manchester, and respondents were asked about aspects of the service or how it was delivered that they found important (Box 7.2). The views of the older people from minority ethnic communities overlapped largely with those of the other groups, with some culturally specific views on what a quality home care service might contain. However, a key finding was that information about the service is not reaching particular communities. As a result, social services departments need to address how they inform people from minority ethnic groups about provision and develop appropriate home care services for them. In addition, the older people in the study talked not only about the care going *into* their home, but also about what happened *outside* it and how this could improve their overall quality of life, including:

Box 7.2: Domiciliary care and older people's priorities

Good quality services need to be organised so that:
- people know what their entitlement is;
- service users are informed if there is to be a change in the carer who is coming to their home;
- carers and their reliefs should be consistent so that trust can be built and time saved;
- the timing of the visit or any change in this is notified to the older person;
- the quality of the services is regularly monitored;
- more domestic cleaning is provided;
- the service can be flexible and what is delivered can reflect the individual's wishes as needs fluctuate. (Raynes et al, 2001, p 69)

- availability of safe accessible and cheap transport;
- getting out of the house;
- improvements in health services;
- good health (Raynes et al, 2001, p 8).

However, as the authors point out, "this is not how home care providers think of home care, nor how services themselves are connected or constructed" (Raynes et al, 2001, p 7). Therefore, they conclude that the development of a quality home care service must actively include other agencies besides social services departments including primary care trusts (PCTs), transportation and the police.

In this, as in other studies (see for example, Godfrey et al, 2000; Tanner, 2001), participants talked about the importance of domestic help as an appropriate task for home carers, even though this is an aspect of home care which is becoming increasingly neglected as social services departments target services towards those people with high intensity needs. Quilgars (2000), in her review of low intensity support services used to help people live independently at home, found no studies on the effectiveness of low-level domiciliary care until a report was written by Clark et al in 1998, commissioned by the Joseph Rowntree Foundation. Entitled '*That bit of help*', this study was based on interviews with 51 older people in three local authority areas, focusing on the value they gave to low-level services, including housework. The study found that the older people made a distinction between *help* (which was designed to assist them in maintaining their independence) and *care* (which they saw as threatening their independence). They regarded housework and other low-level services like gardening and home maintenance as important factors in preventing the need for further care. Women respondents, in particular, valued the contribution that having domestic help made to their own sense of a positive identify and feelings of worth.

Similarly, Tanner (2001), in a small study of 12 older people who had been assessed as ineligible for help from social services found that there was a mismatch between what people felt they needed and what was available, with bathing and cleaning being the two most frequently cited examples. However, when what was deemed as an essential service by social services was refused by the older person, the eligibility criteria were too inflexible to transfer the help into something which they themselves identified as being important:

> Mrs. Anderson had severe osteo-arthritis and continence problems. She preferred to manage her personal care herself, even though it could take her two hours to get washed and dressed in the mornings. She asked social services for help with the heavy cleaning, but was told she could only have help with personal care, which she refused: 'Someone from social services came and said they don't help with cleaning now because no one ever died from having a dirty floor'. (Tanner, 2001, p 118)

The tension between the targeting of resources on people requiring intensive support to remain at home and the recognition of the importance of low-level services that may prevent or delay the need for further care is increasingly apparent. However, as Tanner concludes:

> A measure of effective prevention cannot rest on the narrow basis of cost-effectiveness alone but must encompass psychological and emotional as well as physical well-being. Otherwise, we may succeed in reducing objective indicators of need (such as rates of admission to residential or nursing homes) but at the expense of enabling people to maintain a positive identity. As physical and emotional/psychological well-being are intertwined, only strategies that address both can be deemed effective in the long term. (Tanner, 2001, p 131)

In 2000, Godfrey et al undertook a literature review of the evidence on the effectiveness and outcomes of home care provision in Britain. They found no studies which specifically addressed the issues of the interface between health and social care in the provision of home care services. However, from those studies which looked at the tasks that health and social care staff respectively undertook and how the services were used they were able to conclude that:

- Home care staff increasingly undertake tasks such as supervision of medication and bathing. Community nursing staff have also become more explicit about what constitutes specialist nursing tasks and so what comes within their remit.
- The limited evidence on the extension of social services charging policies identifies that some people are now receiving a service (in particular bathing or respite care) for which they have been means-tested and may be paying, having previously received it free at the point of delivery from a health care provider (Godfrey et al, 2000, p 57).

Throughout the literature on the boundaries between health and social care, a key issue has been the provision of bathing services and which agency should be responsible. Crucial to this discussion is whether the bath in question is a 'health bath' (administered to meet an identified medical need) or a 'social bath' (simply for enjoyment or basic hygiene). Clearly, such a distinction is rarely meaningful for most service users and is based more on attempts to protect limited budgets than on any genuine distinction between the skills or training required to carry out the task in hand.

To some extent, the issue of bathing has always been a matter for discretion. Although it has traditionally been seen as part of the district nurse's role when carried out in conjunction with more technical nursing tasks, bathing as a service in its own right was usually only carried out on an episodic, discretionary basis, fitted in as and when, if at all. Similarly, while the home help service was initially based around the provision of housework and rarely offered personal care, research suggests that some home helps were prepared to offer a degree of intimate care to favoured clients (Twigg, 1997). Following recent changes in the boundaries between health and social care and the increased pressures faced by community services, however, nursing services have tended to retreat without any corresponding advance by social services, leaving the absence of officially defined roles very much exposed to view. Different authorities have responded in different ways, although as the case of Ivy below demonstrates, the presence of an official policy at a local level does not always prevent disputes from occurring.

> Bathing at home has been a perennial area of difficulty within community care. Recurrently described as a 'grey area' of provision, it falls into a territory of ambiguity and uncertainty, caught between the principal service sectors.... Bathing thus lies across the principal fault line of community care: that between the medical and social; and as such, is positioned at the focus of current conflicts within the care system. (Twigg, 1997, pp 211-2)

A similar point is also made by Godfrey et al (2000, p 57) who suggest that:

> The issue of who provides and whether the service is construed as meeting medical or social needs, is intimately bound up with charging policies.

While Ivy's experience of the health and social care divide did not revolve around bathing, it did involve ongoing and heated discussions about a second disputed area where the responsibilities of the health and social care agencies involved were far from clear: the administration of medication.

Ivy's story

Ivy had lived on the ground floor of a sheltered housing project for several years when her physical condition and her memory both began to deteriorate. At first, she began to complain that her eyesight was very limited and that her manual dexterity was so reduced that she had difficulties caring for herself. Later, neighbours reported that she had begun to "wander" round the area at night, looking for a family member who had moved away. As an interim response, the local social services team were able to provide temporary home care support until Ivy could be assessed by a social worker. This case study tells the story of Ivy after the assessment had taken place and the demarcation issues which her case raised for local health and social services.

After Ivy had been assessed by a social worker, it was agreed that she needed help with washing and dressing, preparing meals, taking medication and administering her eye drops. Her GP concluded that her 'wandering' was the result of the fact that she was forgetting to take a sleeping tablet which had been prescribed to overcome longstanding insomnia. When she remembered to take this tablet, she slept soundly throughout the night. When she forgot, she was usually found walking round the area, confused and not sure where she was. Ivy herself recognised that she was becoming confused and said that she wanted support to help her carry on living as independently as possible.

Having identified the issues that needed to be resolved, Ivy, her social worker and the home care organiser met to agree a package to respond to these issues. Everyone present felt that intensive home care support three times a day would be sufficient to help Ivy with her self-care, with her meals and with remembering to take her medication. The only difficulty was her eye drops, which the home care organiser felt was an invasive procedure that could not be performed by an untrained home carer. As a result, a district nurse was contacted with a view to arranging for a nursing input to administer the required eye drops.

After carrying out a separate assessment, the district nurse felt that Ivy was capable of inserting her own eye drops and only needed reminding by her home carer to do so. In contrast, the home care organiser felt that Ivy could not administer the eye drops and that it was against regulations for a home carer to do so on her behalf or even to remind her to do it herself. When Ivy's GP was consulted, he was not sure who was responsible, but emphasised that the drops were crucial to Ivy retaining what little was left of her eyesight. Ivy herself said that she could manage her own drops on a 'good day', but could not tell in advance what was going to be a 'good day' and was worried that she would forget. She also felt that her manual dexterity was so poor that she may slip and injure her eye in the process. Throughout this discussion, both the district nurse and the home care organiser were using the same policy document to support their stance, quoting from a locally agreed, but still controversial, series of job demarcations negotiated by the local authority and local NHS.

At this stage, an impasse was reached and progress seemed difficult to achieve.

When no solution appeared to offer itself, the professionals involved suggested that admission to residential care might be the best thing for Ivy. Ivy herself, who maintained that she was capable of staying where she was if appropriate support was provided, rejected this.

At a second meeting, the situation was much the same. The home care organiser had sought advice from her manager and was told that home carers could not be involved in an invasive procedure, even if only prompting Ivy to take the drops herself. The district nurse remained convinced that it was not a nursing task to remind someone to take eye drops when they were able to insert them themselves. Tensions mounted and a number of heated debates took place between the workers involved, with Ivy present at all times. While the practitioners searched for a solution, Ivy's drops were not being administered at all, thereby jeopardising her remaining eyesight. Being present when those involved in her care were debating who was responsible for looking after her also upset Ivy, who said that it made her feel like a burden and damaged her self-esteem. As a temporary solution, it was eventually agreed that the eye drops would be inserted by Ivy herself with prompts from a home carer while all parties sought further clarification. To make even this concession, the home care organiser had to adapt existing paperwork for oral medication to ensure that this aspect of Ivy's care was properly documented. Six months later, Ivy's condition deteriorated and she was admitted to as nursing home, where her eye drops could be administered under the supervision of nursing staff.

Exercise N: Ivy's story

1. What is your opinion of this situation?
2. How would Ivy have felt during this process?
3. To what extent does Ivy's experience of domiciliary care match that set out by Henwood et al (1998) and Raynes et al (2001) earlier in this chapter?
4. What could have been done differently to achieve a better outcome for Ivy?
5. From your knowledge of local health and social services and from the policy overview in Chapter Three of this book, what new partnership initiatives could have helped to provide more appropriate support for Ivy?

For example:
* *Would a single assessment process help services adopt a more holistic approach to Ivy's needs?*
* *Would an integrated team with a pooled budget provide more appropriate care to people in Ivy's situation?*
* *Would services be able to work more effectively together with a single personal care plan?*
* *Is there scope for closer collaboration between health/social care and housing services?*
* *Which other policies from Chapter Three could help to improve Ivy's experiences in the future?*

Good practice guide

- Be careful where you discuss *demarcation disputes* between health and social services. Debating these issues in front of Ivy only served to increase her distress. What mattered to her was the sort of help she received, not the agency agendas behind how this care would be provided.
- Make sure that the individual service user remains at the *centre of your attention* and practice. In this case, Ivy's eyesight was jeopardised while the various professionals decided whose responsibility it was to administer her eye drops.
- *Listen* to what the service user says and thinks without jumping to conclusions. In this case, Ivy knew that she was becoming confused, that she could manage her eye drops on a 'good' but not a 'bad' day and that there was a risk that she might forget to take them without being reminded. Similarly, she knew that she was capable of staying in her own home with the right support, despite the opinion of those involved that she should enter residential care.
- Try *not to blame* the individuals involved for things which are not their fault. Here, each person had a valid standpoint and was trying their best to provide Ivy with the help she needed. Nobody was being deliberately obstructive; instead, each worker felt constrained by the rules and regulations of their agency. This was no one's fault – it was just a difficult situation wherein those involved had to work to resolve as best they could.

Further reading

For those people interested in the management, effectiveness and outcomes for service users of current domiciliary care services, Godfrey et al (2000) and Sinclair et al (2000) provide comprehensive reviews; in addition, Tanner (2001) provides a fascinating analysis of how a small number of older people managed their needs which were not met by social services and how this was related to their attempts to maintain a positive self-identity. Clark et al (1998) is also a key study on the value of low-level preventative services.

EIGHT

Marjorie's story: older people with mental health problems

If policy debates have traditionally focused on the health and social care divide with regard to institutional care and, more recently, with regard to community services, one group frequently excluded from analysis has been older people with mental health problems. This is to be deeply regretted, not only because the significance of this group of people is growing as a result of demographic changes, but also because they present particular and unique challenges to current single-agency ways of working:

> The care of older people with a mental health problem ... is a major cause for concern and presents a significant challenge for community care.... Social trends show that the number of very elderly people in Britain is increasing, older people are more likely to live alone, and the prevalence of mental ill health rises markedly with age. Therefore, the size of this group is growing and yet it is often forgotten. It is an easy group to ignore. Older mentally ill [people] are reluctant to speak out, are rarely dangerous and are often sad, poor and confused. They may have no family to speak for them. In community care terms, they fall between traditional mental health and older people's services. Their care confronts different professional value systems as a balance is sought between protection and treatment, independence and risk. It requires typically a multi-agency and multi-professional response. Even so, older people with mental health problems are often nobody's priority. (Barnes, 1997, p 1)

Exercise O: Older people with mental health problems

1. How might an older person who is beginning to develop a mental health problem be feeling about the possibility of contacting health/social services and about the future?
2. How might their family be feeling?
3. Are there particular situations or services where the responsibilities of health and social care could overlap?
4. If so, what steps could practitioners and services take to ensure that the services offered to older people with mental health problems are as coordinated as possible?
5. Which of the policies outlined in Chapter Three of this book might help to achieve this goal?

Research findings and service issues

In 1996, research commissioned by the North and South Thames Regional Health Authorities emphasised the scarcity of services for older people with mental health problems (Koffman et al, 1996). Two years previously, a survey of all patients occupying elderly-mentally-ill acute and assessment beds in the two regions had revealed that 368 (24.4%) were inappropriately located and did not require the services provided in a hospital bed. Of these patients, 292 were unable to be discharged home but still needed some form of alternative service provision (ranging from residential care to rehabilitation and from secure inpatient provision to a group home). Of those able to be discharged home, services such as professional support in the home, practical care, more appropriate housing, day care and day hospitals were required. While the study focused primarily on the issue of 'blocked' hospital beds, it did suggest that the reasons alternative services were not being provided was that older people with mental health problems are perceived as being disruptive, requiring high levels of supervision and imposing a heavy workload on staff. In addition, service provision capable of meeting the complex needs of this patient group also tends to be insufficient and under-resourced. The result, in this study, was that the older people concerned were left trapped in hospital with 'no way out'. Koffman et al (1996) contrast this situation with countries like Norway, Holland and France, where they suggest packages of health and social care capable of meeting older people's needs are provided and funded to a more satisfactory level.

Also in 1996, a survey undertaken by the Alzheimer's Disease Society reviewed more than 30 draft continuing care policies to see how much consideration there had been of the needs of people with dementia (cited in George, 1996). Although the Society was only looking for answers to basic questions such as 'Is my relative with dementia able to have NHS continuing care?' and 'Can I get respite from the health service?', it found that most policies were too badly presented and too full of jargon to provide a satisfactory response. Less than half the drafts mentioned dementia at all and only four defined the condition. This omission concerned the Society's executive director, Harry Cayton, who felt that the growing significance of people with dementia should have been recognised.

The following year, the Social Services Inspectorate (SSI) published the results of an inspection of services for older people with dementia in the community in eight local authorities (DoH/SSI, 1997). At the level of frontline practice, the study revealed good working relations, especially where staff were prepared to take a broader view of their role and blur the boundaries of their activities. However, where these arrangements existed, they were often under threat as a result of pressures to define boundaries more clearly and to determine the costs of health and social care. At a strategic level, most social services departments were struggling, and sometimes failing, to work jointly with the NHS. This was especially the case where one agency (usually the social services department) managed its services for people with dementia as part of its services for older people and the other (usually health) as part of its mental health provision. This could result in a situation where the relevant workers from each agency did not know who to speak to in the other service.

Also in 1997, the SSI published a second study based on a workshop for staff and visits to four local authorities (Barnes, 1997). Unlike previous research, the study began with an overview of the incidence of mental health in old age, highlighting both the scale of the current problem and the increasing significance which it will acquire as the older population expands:

- In the 1990s, around 600,000 people in Britain had dementia, and this number is predicted to increase to 900,000 by 2021.
- At any one time, 2-4% of older people are suffering from a major depressive episode and 10-20% from less severe forms of depression.
- Older people accounted for 19% of all suicides in England and Wales in 1992, often linked to depression, pain and feeling unwell. Deliberate self-harm is usually a failed suicide attempt in older people and is associated with serious depression.
- Schizophrenia develops in 1-2% of people aged 65+ and a similar proportion already has the condition before they grow old.
- About 3-4% of older people have an alcohol problem.

These figures are set to increase dramatically as the number of older people increases.

After this broad overview, the report continued with a more detailed analysis of current service issues. Focusing on older people (like Marjorie later in this chapter) with mental health problems and living alone, the report asked why this group of people had traditionally been marginalised by community care services. Key factors included a lack of public concern, difficulties in recognising mental illness in old age and the inability of the group to speak for themselves. However, a major issue was also "the need to cross organisational boundaries in health and social services" (Barnes, 1997, p 9). While the importance of successful multidisciplinary working was emphasised by participants, a number of barriers were identified which could hinder progress:

- The management of services rests with different sectors in health and social services (most are managed with mental health services in the NHS and with older people's services in social services departments).
- Fragmentation of service provision because of budget-led splits and territorial behaviour over health and social care.
- Confusion caused by the complexities of competing health trusts.
- Difficulties in shifting the emphasis from a traditional focus on hospitals to work in the community.
- The lack of co-terminosity of mental health and social services departments.

- The time needed to develop joint strategies as a result of the very low planning and investment base from which work was starting.
- The organisational turbulence experienced by health and social services in recent years.

Despite these, there were efforts at ground level to overcome these obstacles and the importance of flexible joint working was emphasised on a number of occasions:

> During the study visits, stress was placed on the importance of joint work between health and social services so that an integrated service is delivered to the older person. Like books supported by bookends, the care of an older mentally ill person alone can collapse if either side of the support is missing. To maintain this support, a flexible response from both types of services was felt to be crucial. (Barnes, 1997, p 54)

To facilitate greater collaboration, a series of ingredients for successful joint working was identified for those working with older people with mental health problems. Successful joint working:

- need not necessarily be in a team;
- is greatly helped by proximity and professionals knowing each other;
- has developed strongly from joint working over major projects such as the closure of long-stay hospitals;
- can be encouraged by:
  - › liaison with a Department of Old Age Psychiatry, such as monthly meetings in the care management local office;
  - › routine training across health and social service teams;
  - › access to health services professionals (for example, GPs, consultants, community psychiatric nurses [CPNs], occupational therapists [OTs] for social services and vice versa (Barnes, 1997, p 15).

In 1998, further evidence of the marginalisation of older people with mental health problems came from a study of the transition of older patients from acute hospital to continuing institutional long-term care (Cotter et al, 1998). While most patients felt that nobody was listening to them during the discharge process, those with dementia reported that they had not been involved in the discharge process at all. For those with a carer or close friend, it was this person who was consulted, whether or not the person with dementia would have liked to have been involved. Other issues which arose included fragmented and confusing assessment procedures, the lack of choice perceived by users and a lack of attention to people's sense of loss at having to leave their homes. Although staff were aware of many of these issues, they felt powerless to respond, partly as a result of the pressure to maintain a rapid throughput of patients.

In January 2000, the Audit Commission published a report of their review of mental health services for older people in England and Wales. Entitled *Forget me not*, the report was followed up two years later by another study of the same name (Audit Commission, 2002b) which summarised the findings of a series of audits of health and social care mental health services for older people, reviewing how far suggestions for change from the 2000 report had been met (see Box 8.1). The key issue raised by this study is the extent to which recommendations for good practice made in 2000 had not been implemented or followed through by the time of the 2002 study. This raises a significant challenge for frontline practitioners and agencies about the extent to which they feel their services are able to respond to the needs of older people with mental health problems and about what changes are planned to improve practice in this often-neglected area.

More recently, the *National service framework for older people* (DoH, 2001f) has set out new standards for services for older people with mental health problems:

> Older people who have mental health problems [should] have access to integrated mental health services, provided by the NHS and councils to ensure effective diagnosis, treatment and support, for them and their carers. (DoH, 2001f, p 90)

By April 2004, the NHS and councils should have:

- developed local plans with independent sector providers for an integrated mental health service for older people, including mental health promotion;
- agreed protocols used by every general practice to diagnose, treat and care for patients with depression and dementia;
- agreed protocols in place for the care and management of older people with mental health problems. (DoH, 2001f, p 106)

Sadly, the reality of integrated health and local authority services is a far cry from Marjorie's experiences that follow.

Box 8.1: *Forget me not*

Recommendation One
- GPs and other primary care staff should provide information, support and competent advice.

Findings:
- Not all GPs agreed that an early diagnosis of dementia was desirable but nearly all agreed that an early diagnosis of depression was.
- Most carers recalled a physical examination prior to a diagnosis of dementia.
- The majority of GPs did not use assessment scales to aid diagnosis of dementia or depression.

Recommendation Two
- Information about the services available locally, presented in a way that can be understood easily by local people, should be distributed to GP surgeries and other public places.

Findings:
- Once a diagnosis was made, most carers were told what was wrong but fewer were told what to expect.
- About three quarters of carers were told how to access help but a significant number were not.
- Readily available and comprehensive information was only available in a quarter of the areas.

Recommendation Three
- Local mental health professionals should provide training and support for GPs and primary care teams, making particular efforts to contact those who refer very few people.

Findings:
- The majority of GPs had not been trained to diagnose and manage dementia while around two thirds felt they had had sufficient training for depression.
- Few specialist services monitored GP referrals or provided training.

Recommendation Four
- Where possible, assessment should take place by members of a community health team at home on at least one occasion.

Findings:
- Most first assessments were carried out at home.

Recommendation Five
- Provision should be made that is balanced in favour of home-based services.

Findings:
- Home care was not always available out of hours.

Recommendation Six

- A range of specialist community-based staff is needed – ideally with specialist home care workers. Service mangers should consider training home care staff who express an interest in developing skills in this area.

Findings:

- Not all areas had specialist multidisciplinary teams and the mix of professionals varied considerably.
- Few had home care workers trained in mental health.

Recommendation Seven

- Day provision should be made for time-limited assessment and treatment (day hospitals) as well as long-term care (day centres) with an appropriate mix of staff to meet needs. It should be planned jointly by health and social care agencies.

Findings:

- Almost all areas had day hospitals but the scope of their services varied.
- Specialist day centres were less common.

Recommendation Eight

- Respite care should be provided in a range of settings, including at home, with some places reserved for emergency situations.

Findings:

- Fewer than two thirds of carers could get respite care.
- Emergency respite care was available in only half of the areas and home-based care in only a quarter.

Recommendation Nine

- Hospital admission is needed for people with psychiatric and behavioural problems that cannot be managed in any other setting, with close links to physical health care services – with admissions limited by effective community services.

Findings:

- Sometimes people were in hospital because of the lack of community services and hospital facilities were not always suitable for older people with mental health problems.

Recommendation Ten

- Residential and nursing homes are needed, supported by mental health specialists, to enable them to care for highly dependent individuals, with a strong emphasis on quality.

Findings:

- Only two thirds of areas had specialist homes for people with dementia.
- Specialist services provided support and training for homes' staff in only a quarter of areas.

Recommendation Eleven

- NHS-funded continuing care is also required for those in greatest need, as determined jointly by health and social services agencies.

Findings:

- Policies and provision of NHS-funded continuing care varied considerably between areas and, in a third of areas, no comprehensive agreement had been reached.

Recommendation Twelve

- Such complexity requires good coordination between health and social care, with integrated teams of professionals who have ready access to a range of flexible services.

Findings:

- In two fifths of areas most cases were 'jointly worked' between members of the specialist mental health teams.
- In a quarter of areas, specialist teams members were based in the same office.

Recommendation Thirteen

- Effective care planning for individuals is needed, through the Care Programme Approach or a similar method.

Findings:

- Jointly agreed assessment and care management procedures were in place in about a third of areas.
- Key workers were used in nearly all areas.
- Only 6% of areas had culturally appropriate services for older people from minority ethnic groups, although a further half had some limited provision.

Recommendation Fourteen

- Effective information sharing is also needed between practitioners, preferably with shared files.

Findings:

- Shared case files existed in only one tenth of areas, although access to files was available in a further third.
- User or carer held files had not been widely explored.
- Compatible IT systems were available in very few areas.

Recommendation Fifteen

- Clear goals are needed, including the intended balance between home-based, day, outpatient, residential and hospital services.

Findings:

- Nearly half of the areas had clear service goals and plans but a quarter of areas had none.

Recommendation Sixteen
- Good quality information is needed to inform planning, including the monitoring of service quality.

Findings:
- In one third of areas, services were not making full use of demographic data.

Recommendation Seventeen
- A comprehensive service also needs an approach that promotes innovation and works towards jointly commissioned services by health and local authorities, as emphasised by national policy.

Findings:
- Appropriate health and social services personnel were fully involved in joint planning in two thirds of the areas, but people from the voluntary sector, GPs, service users and carers were involved in only half the areas.
- Agencies in just over half the areas were discussing new arrangements for lead purchasing and pooled budgets were in place in about a third of areas.

Source: Adapted from Audit Commission (2000, 2002b)

Marjorie's story

Marjorie was 79 when she first started to experience difficulties swallowing food. At first she could only feel a minor irritation at the back of her mouth, but as time passed she began to sense that there was some sort of blockage starting to grow in her throat. Fearing the worst, she contacted her GP, who referred her to a local hospital for an exploratory operation. Prior to this incident, Marjorie had been an extremely healthy, active person. Friends joked with her that she looked nearer 60 than 80, and she was very outgoing and sociable. As the organist for her local church and a helper at the Sunday school, she used to walk the three miles from her house to the church on a regular basis and enjoyed teaching the children under her supervision. Liked by everyone who knew her, her only regret was that her family, although close emotionally, were some 170 miles away in a different part of the country, keeping in regular contact but visiting only occasionally. This case study tells the story of Marjorie's experience of health and social services after her exploratory operation had taken place and once she had started to develop what her family now believe was a mental health problem.

When Marjorie arrived at the hospital, she was told that her operation would be quite routine – all the doctors needed to do was to remove a sample from the growth in her throat to carry out tests on it. Unfortunately, this was not to be the case, since the growth burst while Marjorie was under anaesthetic, necessitating emergency surgery. This proved successful, and when Marjorie's family arrived, they found her exhausted after her ordeal but, thankfully, alive and apparently well.

As Marjorie's strength began to return she made a very quick physical recovery. Within a few weeks she was ready to go home and hospital staff were amazed at the speed with which she regained her health after so serious an operation. Emotionally and mentally, however, everything was far from all right and her family began to become increasingly concerned about her. To the doctors who had saved Marjorie, she had made a full and very satisfactory recovery. To her family (who knew her before her hospital admission), she was well physically, yet seemed to have suffered some sort of personality change. Instead of the active, outgoing woman who had gone into the operating theatre, they found a person who was not like their mother/grandmother at all – someone who looked about 20 years older, who seemed very depressed and forgetful and who could be quite callous and spiteful. As far as they were concerned, this was a completely different person altogether, and one which they liked a lot less than the Marjorie of old. When they explained these concerns to hospital staff they were told that this was quite normal after a serious operation and that everything would soon return to normal. This seemed like a reasonable explanation, so Marjorie's family tried their best to put their worries from their minds and concentrate on helping her get ready to go home.

When Marjorie was discharged from hospital, it quickly became apparent that everything was anything but 'normal'. Previously very smart and fastidious, Marjorie began to neglect her appearance, failing to wash herself, her clothes or her hair or to flush the toilet after using it. Although her throat had recovered physically, she would not eat or go shopping, and her leftover food began to go mouldy. Refusing to leave the house, she would snap at friends who called round to see her, and began to say very hurtful, personal things to her family.

Now very worried indeed, Marjorie's relatives contacted her GP, who prescribed antidepressants. Although this seemed like a step forward, a neighbour later noticed that Marjorie was simply taking the recommended daily dose out of the packet and hiding it in a small bag down the back of the sofa. At a distance, there was little Marjorie's family could do to help practically. After much discussion, they referred her to social services and tried to arrange for neighbours and a grandson who had recently enrolled at a nearby university to 'keep an eye' on her until a social worker could assess her.

When the social worker called round, she found Marjorie much more capable and alert than she had feared. Marjorie assured her that all she needed was a bit of help with her housework and said that she could not see what all the fuss was about. Her family, in contrast, felt that this was deliberately deceptive behaviour on Marjorie's part, and that she was really much more in need of support than the social worker realised. The social worker made a note of this, but attributed it to the family feeling guilty at being so far away and provided only the support with housework that Marjorie had requested. This included hoovering, dusting and some social stimulation, neglecting to address Marjorie's failure to feed or wash herself properly or the rotting food in her kitchen.

After several weeks, Marjorie was admitted to hospital with severe malnutrition. When the hospital had helped her to regain her strength with 'build-up' drinks, they could find nothing else physically wrong and transferred her to a nearby psychiatric hospital. After a period of assessment, the psychiatric team was unable to find any evidence of a mental health problem that they could diagnose and discharged her home. When the social worker called, Marjorie repeated her plea for help with housework only and her original care package was restored. Throughout this sequence of events, Marjorie's family were in constant communication with the hospital, the psychiatric hospital, the GP and social services, insisting that something was wrong and that Marjorie was not behaving like her old self at all.

With only an occasional visit from a home carer, the burden of caring for Marjorie fell on her elderly neighbours and her grandson, who was sitting exams and was himself undergoing medical tests. Both the neighbours and the grandson felt frustrated with the situation and said that they felt unable to cope.

Several weeks after being discharged home, Marjorie was readmitted to the same hospital with malnutrition. After 'feeding her up' again, the hospital transferred her to the same psychiatric hospital, who carried out another assessment. They were about to discharge her home, when she collapsed and was transferred back to the original hospital for further medical tests. These revealed that Marjorie had developed a secondary cancer from the initial growth in her throat and that nothing further could be done. Preparations were being made to discharge her to a nursing home when she died.

Several years after Marjorie's death her family are still very upset. They believe that Marjorie may have undergone some sort of brain damage during the operation and that she subsequently developed severe depression. They are angry that no one listened to them when they said that Marjorie was not the person she used to be and that she had undergone some sort of personality change. They feel that no one person seemed prepared to take a holistic view of Marjorie's situation and explain to them what might be happening.

The family also feel that none of the services Marjorie received were able to meet her needs, relying too much on the support of her neighbours and grandson and passing her from one agency to another until she died. They claim that this caused unnecessary distress for Marjorie, her neighbours and her family, and wish that she had been spared this anguish by dying when the growth in her throat first burst. Her grandson recalls:

> "In a way, my Gran died when she first went in for the emergency operation. The person who came out wasn't my Gran at all – she was someone else altogether, someone spiteful and not very nice to know. The real Marjorie died in that operating room, but it took months before the matter was finally resolved. During that time something

was clearly wrong, but she didn't seem to meet anyone's criteria and she fell through the hole in the safety net that our health and social services are meant to provide. She just didn't fit in, and in the end they passed her back and forwards until she died."

Exercise P: Marjorie's story

1. What is your opinion of this situation?
2. How would Marjorie and her family have felt during this process?
3. What could have been done differently to achieve a better outcome for Marjorie and her family?
4. From your knowledge of local health and social services and from the policy overview in Chapter Three of this book, what new partnership initiatives could have helped to provide more appropriate support for Marjorie and her family?

For example:

- *Is there scope for local services to develop integrated health and social care for older people with mental health problems using the Health Act flexibilities?*
- *With the advent of user group-specific Care Trusts, is there a danger that older people with mental health problems might fall between mental health and older people's services?*
- *What impact might recent hospital discharge guidance have on the experiences of older people with mental health problems?*
- *How well attuned are new intermediate care services to the needs of older people with mental health problems?*
- *Which other policies from Chapter Three could help to improve the experiences of people like Marjorie in the future?*

Good practice guide

- *Listen to and acknowledge* the contribution of families. They may be right or wrong about the person concerned, but they are often the only ones who know what the older person was like before they became ill. In Marjorie's case, her family had a sense that her change of behaviour and personality was more than a reaction to the operation, but their concerns were not taken seriously by hospital staff.
- *Do not discount people's feelings* and interpretations solely because you think that they are feeling guilty about not providing more support themselves. In this case, the social worker dismissed the family's concerns, attributing them to feelings of guilt at being so far away.
- *Do not exploit neighbours and family members* or take their contribution for granted. Here, Marjorie's neighbours and grandson felt a tremendous sense of responsibility for her which in the end became too much.

- Try to find a solution that meets a person's needs without pigeonholing them into a particular category. Try also to respond by looking at the *whole of the person's situation*, not just at the aspects that your agency has traditionally dealt with. In this case, Marjorie's needs did not fit the remit of any of the agencies involved and she was transferred between an acute hospital, a psychiatric hospital and social services until she died.

Further reading

The two Audit Commission reports (2000, 2002b) give a comprehensive overview of the current state of mental health services for older people. Also included in *Forget me not* (Audit Commission, 2000) are some detailed case studies of good practice or service development initiatives in England and Wales.

Also useful is the SSI's work on older people and mental health (Barnes, 1997; DoH/SSI, 1997) and the government's blueprint for the way forward in the *National service framework for older people* (DoH, 2001f). Details of the *National service framework for older people* can be found at the Department of Health's website (www.dh.gov.uk/PolicyAndGuidance/HealthAndSocialCareTopics/).

NINE

Mary and Dennis' story: primary care

Following the changes announced in *Shifting the balance of power* (DoH, 2001j; see Chapter Three of this book), primary care is increasingly becoming the focus for partnership working between health and social care. However, this is a relatively recent development and most partnership working between health and social care has traditionally tended to take place between social services departments and former health authorities, with primary and community health services having little input (Rummery and Glendinning, 2000). As primary care is taking on a much greater role, however, a number of different models have been developed to promote greater collaboration at both operational and strategic levels. Examples include GP-attached social workers, integrated teams, social services representatives on former primary care group (PCG) boards and now primary care trust (PCT) executives and, most recently, representation in new Care Trusts. Despite this, research to date suggests that there are still a number of barriers to closer partnership working, including a lack of shared boundaries, different contractual arrangements between different workers and different professional values (see, for example, Wistow et al, 1997; Rummery and Glendinning, 2000). In addition, there is a danger that recent reorganisations of healthcare in particular may hinder rather than strengthen partnership working as boundaries alter and key members of staff change roles.

After reviewing the research findings, this chapter tells the story of Mary and Dennis, who were able to gain access to preventative services and stave off a potential crisis due to early contact with a GP-attached social worker.

Exercise Q: Primary care

1. Primary care includes a range of community health services such as general practice, district nursing and health visiting: how much use do older people make of these services and how important is primary care as a location for meeting the needs of older people?
2. Are there particular situations or services where the responsibilities of health and social care could overlap?
3. If so, what steps could practitioners and services take to ensure that the services offered to older people are as coordinated as possible?
4. Which of the policies in Chapter Three of this book might help to achieve this goal?

Research findings and service issues

As Poxton (1999) observes, most of the links between primary healthcare and social services since the community care reforms of the 1990s have involved joint working (day-to-day partnership working in operational settings) rather than joint commissioning (the strategic joint commissioning of services). With regard to the former, there are a number of models, including social workers based in GPs surgeries, one-stop shops and integrated teams, but fewer examples of collaboration at strategic levels which have resulted in significant changes in the configuration of services for older people. Much of the research reviewed later in this chapter includes schemes which were in place either before the creation of PCGs in April 1999 or PCTs in April 2002, and the potential impact of these new organisations on the health and social care divide is still unclear. Nevertheless, lessons can be learnt from early schemes to inform future collaboration between primary care and social services.

Joint working

Prior to the community care reforms of the 1990s, there were examples of care management schemes which involved social workers working with health professionals in primary care settings (reviewed in Challis, 1999). There were few guidelines for the implementation and management of such projects which were often the results of the combined innovative efforts of GPs and local social services teams who had traditionally had good working relationships (see, for example, Walters, 2001).

Indeed, much of the early research on joint working involved the evaluation of small-scale projects of social workers attached to or located within GPs surgeries. The findings were largely positive, reporting improved liaison between GPs and social workers, more appropriate referrals to social workers, faster responses by them but often a substantial increase in workloads because of earlier intervention (see, for example, Cumella, 1994). More recent evaluations have attempted to identify what makes collaboration work and the organisational implications for health and social services of extending this way of working (see, for example, Cumella et al, 1996; Le Mesurier and Cumella, 1996, 2001).

Describing the findings of case studies in four different locations of social care workers linked to, or based within, GP practices during the mid-1990s, Rummery and Glendinning (2000) identify the main benefits and disadvantages for the key players (Box 9.1).

Despite the obvious advantages for many of the key players, Rummery and Glendinning (2000, p 72) identify three main reasons why many such schemes remained short-term projects and have not been widely transferred (see page 132).

Box 9.1: GP-attached social work

Local and health authority managers' perspectives:
- Schemes appear to offer comparable services at no increased cost and may result in fewer emergency admissions to hospital and less use of expensive institutional care.
- Costs to social services appear to be higher (and benefits lower) in terms of changes to working practices than for health professionals.

Primary care professionals' perspectives:
- Primary health professionals identified the most significant benefits as quicker access to social services, fewer delays, less frustration as a result of improved communication and better understanding between the professions.
- Community nurses were rarely involved in the development of schemes but reported improved communication, reduced delays in referrals and better feedback.
- There are some reports of improved health outcomes for patients but this was not borne out by quantifiable evidence.
- Some GPs perceived a reduction in patients attending surgery for social rather than health reasons.
- Unrealistic expectations at the outset meant that social services could not always provide what primary care professionals would have liked.
- Schemes could not improve services available to patients or overcome budgetary limitations.

Social care workers' perspectives:
- Some schemes resulted in improved job satisfaction due to improved interprofessional working and increased autonomy.
- There were significantly higher workloads for GP-attached social workers than for colleagues in area teams.
- Most reported increased isolation, either because of inadequate supervision from their manager, a lack of awareness or unrealistic expectations of their role by health professionals, or a feeling of being caught between two agencies.
- There were greater changes to working practices required from them and this was not always acknowledged or appreciated by healthcare workers.

Patients' perspectives:
- Easier and often quicker access to a named worker without bureaucracy of social services.
- No stigma associated with accessing social services through primary care.
- No evidence of improvement in quantity or quality of services.
- No patient involvement in design of schemes, therefore their preferences often not addressed. (Adapted from Rummery and Glenndinning, 2000, pp 67-72)

- many have been set up using time-limited project money;
- participants did not fully anticipate or acknowledge the particular barriers to collaboration in primary care;
- benefits to all parties have not been seen to be equally distributed and many social services departments were unwilling to sustain the schemes.

While the co-location of social care workers and primary healthcare workers may be one way to assist collaboration between professionals, it is not the only prerequisite. In 1997, Tucker and Brown published the results of a study in which they compared the benefits and effectiveness of three different models of providing community care services in Wiltshire:

1. Traditional social services adult care teams working separately from Primary Health Care Teams (PHCTs) but collaborating as necessary on individual cases.
2. Social services and the health authority jointly funding link workers based in GP surgeries. The link workers may be nurses, social workers or occupational therapists (OTs) but were employed by the social services department and accessed their budget through the adult care team manager.
3. Social services and PHCTs establishing joint health and social care teams to provide an integrated service for patients from two GP practices. Individual team members were managed by their own agencies and held separate budgets.

The results of the study showed that there was no obvious difference between the three models in terms of the speed of response to referrals or the type of care provided to service users. Nevertheless, there was a greater confidence from referrers to the link workers and integrated teams that better communication meant that referrals would not get "swallowed up into an impersonal 'duty system' and get lost" (Tucker and Brown, 1997, p 17). The proximity of link workers and integrated team members meant that getting in touch with other professionals was much easier and more joint assessment and planning went on between health staff and social workers here than from adult care teams. Even so, where adult social workers had cases which were complex and required significant input from both agencies, the will to work together was apparent.

The link workers, who were physically separate from other social services workers, often had to work more flexibly than their counterparts in adult care teams. While all the link workers interviewed reported a good relationship with their PCHT, some expressed feelings of isolation:

> I often feel like piggy in the middle between the two services ... having to hear [each service] say bad things about the other. (Tucker and Brown, 1997, p 23)

Others factors inhibited the potential for joint working. The most apparent was the lack of shared budgets and incidents where there was 'cost-shunting' between the two agencies over individual patients. Second, where there was a lack of clarity about the roles of different professionals in the integrated teams, good team working was hindered. For example, the role of the district nurse was ambiguous – in theory they could be care managers and carry out social care assessments, but in practice some were anxious about that role. Similarly, some social workers felt that their roles had changed to become more medically orientated.

Also in 1997, the Nuffield Institute for Health published some results from their sub-study on links between primary healthcare and social services (Wistow et al, 1997). Having examined the experiences of five localities across England, the study identified long-standing problems related to organisational, operational, professional and cultural issues, but also evidence of innovative and imaginative practice where joint working and commissioning were working well. In particular, this report identifies some general themes from all the sites, analysing them in a way which demonstrates how different localities dealt with some of the common issues which arose:

- *Organisational shift versus individual entrepreneurialism:* individual 'champions of change' were often found in the study sites, either having emerged or been appointed. In either case, the problem of relying on individuals to initiate change rather than interagency agreements is that when individuals move, initiatives flounder.
- *Excellence versus equity:* the problem of allocating scarce resources across the localities was well understood. Typically, where there were too few social workers to be attached to all GPs surgeries that were interested in such arrangements, or where some practices expressed more interest than others, there was felt to be little alternative but to pursue excellence for some at the expense of equity.
- *Cost versus benefit:* all localities were aware that primary care/social care collaboration was time-consuming and that effort put into this area would inevitably reflect in a cost elsewhere.
- *Medical/nursing versus social models:* while the study found evidence of cultural barriers between health and social care professions based largely on different value bases, it also found other evidence that showed, where social workers were working effectively within GPs surgeries, these barriers had been overcome.
- *Flexibility versus agreements:* although it was generally agreed that there needed to be broad guidelines about structuring relationships between professionals from primary health and social care, in practice, where there had been pilot projects of social workers in GPs surgeries, in most cases there were no formal agreements about roles and responsibilities. Instead, these had been left to evolve and develop.

- *Project management versus mainstream management:* how new projects were managed was a key issue. The study came across examples of projects which had faltered once the funding for the project manger had ceased. The report advocates the careful evaluation of whether innovations need special management or whether existing without such support is the key test of its success.
- *Co-location versus non-co-location:* there was strong agreement that co-location was the preferred model for joint working in order to aid communication and improve access for service users. However, as previously identified, there were problems in allocating too few social workers to too many practices and difficulties for social services in reconciling that model with existing geographical boundaries and client specialisms.
- *Team loyalty versus organisational loyalty:* where integrated team members are employed by different organisations, there is a potential for split loyalties. In this study, this was particularly a dilemma for social workers based within health teams who may feel exposed to different expectations from two different agencies.
- *Social work versus care management:* there was some confusion about the role of the social worker within the health setting. Should workers be undertaking traditional social work (working in a more preventative way and giving emotional and psychological support to patients) or acting as care managers (focusing on crisis intervention and carrying out community care assessments)? In particular, it was often assumed that practice-based social workers would be able to work with people who would not usually be seen by social workers. While this offered greater scope for prevention, it also takes resources away from those people in most need.
- *Markets versus hierarchies versus networks:* those initiatives in the study which had done most to establish good collaboration between primary health and social services were based on a model of networks, characterised by cooperation and equality, rather than formal agreements and hierarchies.

Between August 1998 and March 1999, the Social Services Inspectorate undertook an inspection of links between social services and primary health services in eight authorities, looking at the state and quality of joint working in older people's services (O'Hagan, 1999). They found a wide range of small-scale partnerships which offered good quality services to older people. However, there was concern that successful projects had not become common practice within social services and that:

> These successes were the exceptions that operated in a context of social services and primary health services for older people working in parallel lines rather than in partnership. (O'Hagan, 1999, p 12)

In addition, the Social Services Inspectorate (SSI) identified a number of lessons to be learned from the successful partnerships and key messages to assist development (Box 9.2).

Box 9.2: Lessons from successful partnerships

- Users benefit from services that are more responsive through being more integrated.
- Community nurses are frequently the most active participants in primary health care teams in linking with social services. Social services need to focus on this when developing more joined up practice with primary health services.
- Partnership-orientated funding arrangements have acted as an important stimulus for partnership work. The new arrangements for joint working with the NHS created by the Health Act 1999 can be used to make a difference.
- Strong relationships between practitioners and professionals are at the heart of success.
- There is a rich range of models of good practice for social services departments to use to increase their understanding of joint working and consider as a basis for further development.
- Small-scale worthwhile partnerships do not by themselves usually generate a momentum to roll out more widely. (O'Hagan, 1999, pp 2, 12)

Much of the research identified above has focussed on the process of joint working between primary healthcare and social services. But, "the real test of services is not how smoothly the process runs, but whether or not individuals are better off through contact with them" (Henwood and Waddington, 2000, foreword). With this in mind, the Department of Health commissioned the Outcomes of Social Care for Adults (OSCA) research initiative (summarised in 2000 in a report by the Nuffield Institute for Health) (Henwood and Waddington, 2000). The report describes the findings of 13 projects focusing on the outcomes of services for users, one of which investigated the consequences of co-locating health and social care staff, particularly for older people and their carers.

The study took place in two London boroughs with contrasting arrangements for partnership working between primary health and social care. Area One had moved its adult care teams into health centres with community nurses, while Area Two had five teams in community care centres, not co-located with GPs or community nurses. The sample included 224 older people aged 75+ who were eligible for community care assessments. The research collected data by a range of quantitative and qualitative methods, including interviews with older people and their carers and establishing outcomes for the older people in terms of whether they were still in the community or in institutional care six months after the initial interview. Overall, the main finding was that the different arrangements for collaboration between primary care and social care staff was not a key determining factor in whether or not the older people remained at home six months after assessment. What was most significant was:

• the level of the older people's cognitive functioning (measured by the Mini Mental State Examination);
• the number of home care hours per week.

Other findings were that:

• satisfaction with services was not related to forms of collaboration between health and social care;
• collaboration with the older person is more important than communication about them between professionals.

The study concluded:

> On the basis of this study in two areas, we have insufficient evidence to support or refute a policy of full-scale co-location of social and primary care, on grounds of a link between the arrangements for collaboration and its outcomes for older people. The quality and effectiveness of communication with clients may be determined in part by the quality of communication between professionals and in part by other factors, including the skills and knowledge of individual practitioners. This needs further exploration before assumptions are made about the benefits of any setting or mode of working to the process of care delivery and its outcomes. (Henwood and Waddington, 2000, p 124)

More recently, research into frontline collaboration between primary care and social care workers has compared outcomes for older people from integrated health–social care teams and traditional social work teams in Wiltshire (Brown et al, 2002, 2003). The integrated teams comprised social workers, social work assistants, OTs, OT assistants and district nurses who were all located in large fundholding practices (replaced by PCGs in April 1999). The sample group comprised 393 people who had been referred to social services via the integrated teams or the traditional teams for a community care assessment between July 1999 and June 2000. The findings from this research have significant implications for the future development of collaboration of primary care and social services:

• There was no difference between the two models in the proportion of people who were living independently 18 months after the initial referral.

- Patients from the integrated teams were more likely to be referred by themselves or their family. This may suggest that health professionals are becoming more familiar with the roles of social care workers and are recommending that patients request their help and/or that patients are more at ease with the notion of seeking help from social services staff within the GP surgery. Furthermore, the speed of response from referral to assessment was slightly faster in integrated teams. These two findings indicate that the 'one-stop' shop approach can be useful for accessing services, particularly within rural communities.
- A greater proportion of the integrated group went into residential care over the 18-month period. This may be explained by a slightly older age profile and a greater degree of depression, but Brown et al (2003, p 93) also speculate that "it could be that higher admission rates to residential care might be an unintended consequence of integrated teams where a more 'medical model' might begin to predominate".
- Comparison of the relative costs of service delivery between the two groups was complex and incomplete. A partial analysis of available data suggested that the traditional approach appeared more cost–effective, but no firm conclusions were drawn.
- The older people had little interest in who organised or delivered their services as long as the care provided met their needs. There were no differences in their levels of satisfaction.
- Older people in both groups had experienced difficulties in accessing services for various reasons including difficulty in getting information, not knowing who to contact and confusion around eligibility.
- The importance of the relationship between the older people and service providers, and in particular their home carers, was highlighted by many respondents.

In particular, this research suggests that locating social services and health staff within integrated teams may not be more clinically effective for older people than traditional methods of service delivery. It concludes that the degree of integration of the teams examined may have improved the process of seeking help and communication between professionals, but is insufficient to have any real effect on the outcomes of care for the older people.

Overall, the evidence from the research about the benefits for service users and patients of joint working between primary health and social services is at best inconclusive. Despite this, Rummery and Glendinning (2000, p 78) summarise a number of the key lessons about partnership working from previous joint projects (Box 9.3).

Box 9.3: Partnership working in primary care

- The commitment of key managers and budget holders in both organisations is necessary for sustainable collaboration.
- Collaboration needs to have benefits for both parties involved; the costs of collaboration should not be borne unequally by one side.
- Participants need to have realistic, achievable goals.
- The roles and responsibilities of participants need to be clearly understood at the outset.
- It is particularly important to ensure that community nurses are fully involved.
- The barriers to interorganisational and interprofessional collaboration need to be acknowledged and addressed.
- Patients need to be involved to ensure that plans reflect their needs and priorities. This is unlikely to happen without sufficient development support.
(Rummery and Glendinning, 2000)

Strategic issues

Following the community care reforms there were some early attempts at joint commissioning between social services and primary care, the results of which have relevance for future strategic development. For example, Poxton (1999) describes the King's Fund Joint Commissioning Project which ran from 1996 to 1998. Five sites across England were involved in a variety of different approaches to primary health and social care partnerships. While there were many examples of joint working in the projects, there were far fewer examples of more strategic joint collaboration. Key themes from this research include (Poxton, 1999, pp 2–3):

- *Joint commissioning and GP practices*: while there were some attempts to jointly assess the needs of individual patients and jointly plan care packages, there was no real evidence of any identification of needs of practice populations or planning of services around individual practices or group of practices. Restrictions around budgets made any major changes to services impossible.
- *Joint commissioning and locality groups*: in the five sites, health and social care had been involved together in locality groups for between six months and two years. There was some evidence of health and social services managers working together but efforts were focused on improving existing working practices or securing funding for new small-scale projects.
- *Service outcomes*: specific outcomes could be identified for individual patients where health and social care professionals had worked together, but locality groups had little power to affect the major configuration of services.

- *Political process*: joint working had proved most effective where the complexity and sensitive nature of the task had been recognised. Clear vision, leadership and development support across boundaries was crucial.
- *Decision making*: a clear knowledge of who is doing what and responsibility and powers around decision making is critical for effective joint commissioning. Unfortunately this was not always apparent in the development sites. At both practice and agency levels, differences in working styles and procedures made joint decision making difficult. There was also evidence of weak links between decisions made at practice, locality and strategic levels and a poor flow of communication between them.
- *Budgets*: difficulties caused by different financial planning cycles and lack of capacity to pool resources were a major impediment to successful joint commissioning. Changes to the configuration of services in the projects were therefore only small.
- *Engaging users and carers*: in only one of the development sites, where user and carer involvement was already established, was there any evidence of local people being involved in discussions about the delivery and development of services. Here, user and carer involvement ensured that the partnership responded to the needs of the population and did not focus solely on the working practices of the professionals. Elsewhere, there appears to have been too much concern about the nature of these relationships to involve users and carers at the early stages of partnership working.

In 1999, the SSI (O'Hagan, 1999) found some improvement in the experiences of agencies attempting to undertake joint commissioning as some of the difficulties identified earlier (particularly budgetary constraints) had been eased. However, "there was little evidence of joint strategic work to create an overall more integrated approach between social and primary health care services" (O'Hagan, 1999, p 14). On a positive note, the representation of social services on PCG boards had raised primary care up the social services agenda. This contribution was valued, although the report concluded that the effectiveness of this involvement would in part depend on representatives' place in their departmental management structure. Generally, there was little evidence of the two agencies working together to identify the needs of the older population and to begin to develop and implement long-term community care services (although this was beginning to be achieved through work on local Joint Investment Plans; see Chapter Three of this book). For the most part, however, the lessons from small pilot projects which were good examples of effective partnership working had not been applied more generally across health and social care agencies.

More recent research on the state of partnership working between social services and PCG/Ts is reported in the *National tracker survey of primary care groups and trusts* (a three-year longitudinal survey of a nationally representative sample of 72 PCGs established in 1999). The final study, covering 2001/2002 (Wilkin et al,

2002), identifies a number of key findings with regard to services for older people. This has been summarised by Coleman and Glendinning (2002) (Box 9.4).

Box 9.4: Partnership working and the National Tracker Survey

Strategic planning:
- The role of social services representatives on PCG boards/PCT executives as a strategic link between the two agencies was developing slowly.
- There was a high turnover of social services representatives, with half of those surveyed thinking that geographical boundary issues continued to create barriers.
- The use of modernisation grants for joint health/social services service developments had increased steadily since 1999/2000.
- Just over half (55%) of the PCG/Ts were reported to be involved in local initiatives using Health Act flexibilities.
- Only a minority of PCG/Ts had completed mapping of existing services with social services and identified the need for new service provision.
- 70% of PCG/Ts had appointed staff to develop partnerships with local authorities, and 58% had jointly appointed coordinators to develop intermediate care services.

Operational level:
- Joint training activities had taken place in 89% of PCG/Ts.
- Changes in health and social services workforce (including reorganisation and relocation of staff, secondments and transfers) were reported in 89% of PCG/Ts.
- Two fifths of social services representatives said there were co-location or links between GPs and social services staff in the area.
- However, 48% reported difficulties in trying to improve collaboration between PCG/T and local authority staff, with changes in terms and conditions of employment being the most difficult to negotiate.
- Joint commissioning was taking place in 78% of PCG/Ts, the most common services being community-based rehabilitation schemes and intermediate care services.
- Progress in implementing the single assessment process appeared slow, with nearly half the social services representatives having little knowledge of its implementation.
- Integrated care management was developed, fully or partially, in two fifths of the PCG/Ts.
- Problems in discharging older people from hospital were reported by nearly two thirds of social services representatives.

Wider partnership networks:
- The majority (90%) of chief executives reported regular meetings with senior local authority colleagues other than social services.
- All PCG/Ts were working with community regeneration, 80% with leisure and 77% with housing.
- All PCG/Ts reported being involved in at least one multi-agency, locally based initiative.
- More flexible funding had allowed many PCG/Ts to redirect some of their resources into non-traditional (and non-NHS) initiatives aimed at improving health or quality of life.
- Partnerships with private sector organisations had increased slightly since 2000/01 but nearly a half still reported no such activity. (Adapted from Coleman and Glendinning, 2002)

In summary, it is clear that partnership working between primary care and social services is now high on the agenda of both agencies. Despite longstanding emphasis on the need to develop closer relationships between health and social care, the opportunities for new ways of working and developing new services for older people allowed by recent legislative changes are only now being explored. The research evidence on models of joint working between frontline staff suggests that there may be benefits in terms of improved communication and liaison, and improvements for older people in terms of the process of accessing services, but no significant improvements in terms of outcomes of care. Nevertheless, the perceived benefits for older people of accessing social care services via the health services should not be underestimated, as the account of Mary and Dennis' experiences show.

Mary and Dennis' story

Mary (77) and Dennis (75) have been married for 50 years and have spent most of that time living in a privately rented house. They have a son, Graham (48), who retired early on health grounds and who lives nearby with his wife. They have two married children. Mary and Dennis also have a daughter, Brenda (40), living locally, who works full time and spends one day a week away from home. Her husband is also in full-time employment and they have two children aged six and 10.

Throughout their lives, both Mary and Dennis have kept in reasonably good health and only two years ago begun to visit their GP more regularly – Mary for varicose veins and Dennis for a series of dizzy spells for which he was prescribed medication. At that point the GP suggested that the couple both applied for Attendance Allowance and referred them to the local social services department as he thought they could do with "that extra bit of help" now that they were becoming increasingly infirm. Mary and Dennis have always been deeply suspicious of social workers and, after the first and only visit, asked them not to call again, assuring them that they could mange. They did all their own housework and laundry, and despite Mary's increasingly poor mobility, they did most of their shopping on public transport. Family members helped out willingly where necessary. Mary and Dennis applied successfully for Attendance Allowance and they continued to live their lives without assistance from any caring agencies for the next two years. Efforts by the family to get them to consider moving to smaller ground-floor accommodation met with no success.

During that time Mary and Dennis' GP retired and was replaced by a doctor whom they grew to like and trust. She referred Mary to the hospital where she was diagnosed with glaucoma and visited them at home when necessary. The couple visited the practice nurse yearly for their over-75 check and flu jabs, but Dennis rarely had occasion to see the GP. Despite complaining more regularly of dizzy spells, he refused to visit the GP when they happened. During this time, the family noticed that Dennis was getting more forgetful, occasionally repeating the same question several times, but the couple appeared to be managing reasonably well and continued to get out and about.

A week before Easter, Mary suddenly became unwell. She felt exhausted and lethargic and unable to get out of bed. Graham visited his parents every day, preparing food and organising shopping. Brenda took over at the weekend. This entailed taking Dennis to her house in order to let Mary rest. During this time it became apparent that Dennis' short-term memory was very poor – the shock of Mary's illness seemed to have thrown him into confusion and he had difficulty remembering faces and names and needed total supervision of all domestic activities within the home. The doctor visited and prescribed medication for Mary but also suggested that she ask the social worker based within the GP practice to visit the couple, feeling that now was the time for them to receive some domiciliary support. Graham was very reluctant to have a social worker visit as he had recently had experience of another local social services department which had provided assistance to his mother-in-law, Alice, before her admission to residential care. They had encountered a number of problems including:

- having to repeat basic information to three people on the phone before a social worker visited and took the same information;
- waiting five days for a social worker to visit despite feeling that the situation was critical and required immediate attention;
- duplicating information to a district nurse who visited at the request of the GP;
- being misled about the availability and timing of calls to help his mother-in-law get up and go to bed;
- having to wait six days between the initial assessment and domiciliary services actually starting while the social worker rang a number of private agencies to ascertain availability and secure funding;

- finding that the message book system that had been set up in the house for all care workers to communicate with each other was not being used;
- unreliability of carers arriving;
- experiencing six different carers for as many calls in three days;
- finding requests by the family about, for example, making sure Alice had clean clothing, had been ignored;
- having a different social worker organising the admission to a residential home from the one who did the initial assessment and arranged services at home.

It was a surprise to Graham, therefore, that his mother agreed to a social worker visiting, but she felt confident in the GP and saw it as an extension of the service they got from the surgery. By that time, Mary's condition had deteriorated and the GP diagnosed Mary as having had a slight stroke. Mary was confined to bed and Graham was spending all day at their house, offering total personal care for his mother but also keeping his father occupied. The whole family feared that Mary would be taken into hospital (a possibility she fiercely resisted) but were certain that Dennis could not stay at home alone. Mary was adamant that Dennis should not go into residential care so Graham offered to have him stay with him and/or Brenda. With a Bank Holiday coming up they were not at all hopeful of any home-based services being available. However, his parents' experiences could not have been more different from that of his mother-in-law:

- the practice-based social worker arrived the day after the GP had requested the visit;
- she arrived with all the basic information to hand and it was accurate;
- before visiting she had talked with the GP and agreed that Mary was eligible for the 'Hospital at Home' scheme, a new service jointly commissioned by social services and the PCT designed to prevent people being admitted to hospital;
- while she assessed Mary's needs primarily, she noted how interdependent the couple were and that, without Mary, Dennis could not manage alone;
- she recognised immediately that Dennis was either experiencing an acute confusional state or the early stages of dementia;
- as well as seeking Mary and Dennis' views, she spoke to Graham and Brenda to see how they perceived the situation and also how they were affected by the change in their parents' circumstances;
- the social worker quickly gained the whole family's commitment to work with her in putting together a suitable package of services. Mary felt most uncomfortable with her children providing personal care for her and so the priority was to free them from these tasks.

Once back at the health centre, the social worker accessed the 'Hospital at Home' scheme and arranged two visits a day, one in the morning (when two carers visited to get Mary washed, dressed and out of bed, and to supervise Dennis getting up and dressed and assist him getting their breakfasts) and one in the evening (where one carer assisted them both getting to bed). The carers monitored Mary's physical condition, calling in the GP on one occasion when her temperature rose dramatically. As this was primarily a health resource, there was no charge for this service. In addition, the social worker arranged a home carer from a private agency to go in at lunchtime and teatime to serve food which had been prepared by family members. As Mary and Dennis were in receipt of Attendance Allowance, they paid a set rate for this service. With Mary and Dennis' permission, the social worker talked to the GP about Dennis' condition and, once the GP had ruled out any acute infection which may have led to the confusion, she referred him to a psycho-geriatrician.

Members of the family visited daily but the social worker arranged additional support from a befriending service run by a local voluntary dementia group. A carer from this initiative visited twice a week and took Dennis on the bus to go shopping and helped him at home to continue to do the jobs he was physically able to do but needed supervision to complete.

After a month, Mary's health improved. At a review, the social worker and family agreed on a new package of care. It no longer involved the 'Hospital at Home' service, but a home carer continued to call twice a day to undertake an agreed range of tasks. This allowed Mary and Dennis to continue to live interdependently, but relieved Mary of some of the responsibility of being the main carer of her husband (who was now diagnosed with dementia). Again the couple paid a set rate for this service as it was not a health resource, but this had been explained to them in advance of the review and Mary was more than happy to pay as she regarded the service as critical in enabling them both to live at home. The carer from the dementia group continued to visit Dennis and the social worker agreed to find out about other services that might be available as his condition deteriorated.

Six months later, the couple were still living at home and, as well as receiving home-based services, Dennis was attending day care twice a week at a residential home and was about to have his first week of respite care there.

Exercise R: Mary and Dennis' story

1. What is your opinion of this situation?
2. What service are people more likely to get in your area – that offered to Alice or that offered to Mary and Dennis?
3. How would Mary and Dennis have felt during this process?

Good practice guide

- *Prepare well* for initial assessments. People are reassured when professionals act quickly, are well informed and demonstrate that they have talked with other relevant people.
- Older people sometimes initially feel embarrassed about talking to social workers but often feel less anxious about talking to a worker from the health centre. *Try to imagine what the person you are visiting may be feeling.*
- *Do not make assumptions about the kind of help that people might want* and try to arrange services flexibly in order to meet the needs that people identify themselves. In this situation, Mary preferred having paid workers coming in to do personal things for them rather than their own children. It was less embarrassing and they were properly trained to do lifting and moving. Other people may take exactly the opposite view of the same situation.
- *Do not make assumptions about what family members or people who have been offering care in the past are able to do in the future.* In this case, although Graham and Brenda did not have to come and get their parents up, put them to bed or serve food, they visited as frequently, brought the children to visit and resumed some of the social interaction with them which had been completely lost before paid carers took over.
- Take the time to *listen to people* and their families about what they want and pay attention to the detail they tell you. They will all be able to help construct a care plan which is more likely to work if all parties have contributed to it.
- Make sure that any services that are arranged are *reliable*, arrive as agreed and, where possible, that there is *continuity* in the carers.
- Find the *most suitable way to communicate* with all the people who are likely to be visiting, whether they be carers or friends or family. A message book in the person's home is only useful if everyone knows it is there and uses it.

Further reading

Primary care is now a key site for a range of partnership activities. Key sources include DoH (2001j), which summarises the role that primary care is now playing within health and social care; Poxton (1999); and Rummery and Glendinning (2000). For further information about the work of individual PCTs, see www.nhs.uk

TEN

Postscript: Sid and May's story

In spite of New Labour's stated commitment to bringing down the 'Berlin Wall' between health and social services, the reality for practitioners in the field is that effective joint working remains problematic. Across a range of services, different cultures, policies, agendas, funding priorities, administrative systems and legal requirements all have the potential to make the day-to-day experience of interagency collaboration extremely frustrating, time-consuming and, all too often, unsuccessful. In the early 21st century, the policy context is constantly evolving and there is no sign that this process is drawing to a close. Following the election of a New Labour government in May 1997, indeed, the rate and pace of change has increased substantially, and it may well be that further reform is imminent.

Whatever the future holds, however, this book has sought to provide a human face to the administrative, legal and bureaucratic difficulties of joint working between health and social services. For people like Andrew, Bert, Babu, Ben, Ivy, Marjorie, Mary and Dennis, the most important thing is receiving high quality services that meet their needs. Who actually provides the services and the demarcation disputes which can arise are issues for workers to resolve and, in an ideal world, should not impinge on individual service users at all. In reality, of course, this is often not the case, and the failure of health and social care agencies to provide a coordinated response can add to, rather than resolve, service users' difficulties, generating feelings of anger, indignation, betrayal and exhaustion. This is often not the fault of the practitioners involved, who themselves feel frustrated and restrained by the various barriers to interagency working. However, the fact remains that individuals are not receiving the services they need because of artificial and service-led divisions between health and social care.

If readers take only one message away from this book, it is that the problematic nature of the health and social care divide can impact negatively on the lives of individual service users and that workers need to be sufficiently informed and flexible to reduce as much of this impact as they can. While 'the Wall' still stands, this seems the most positive way forward.

Of course, in writing this book we have tended to present each of the key chapter headings as if they are separate issues. In practice, however, this is often not the case, and there is considerable scope for the problems associated with areas of provision such as domiciliary care, intermediate care, hospital discharge and mental health to combine, interact and compound each other. As an illustration of this, we end with Sid and May's story – a real-life account of what happened to a real-life older couple when the services involved in their care were not able to provide a sufficiently holistic and person-centred package of services.

Sid and May's story

Since 1947, Sid (84) and May (85) had lived in a house rented from a charitable trust in a suburban area of an English city. They had both worked for a local firm and retired in their sixties with modest works pensions. Their children, who were 59 and 50, lived locally; the family saw a lot of each other, visiting each other and going out to local restaurants for meals with their extended family.

Until recently, May and Sid were both relatively healthy, but Sid's arteries in his legs were hardening and he had difficulty walking more than a few hundred yards. He used a walking stick, but for some years did all the cooking, housework and family finances. In 1986, he had a minor stroke, but made a full recovery.

May was very fit, being capable of walking quite long distances unaided. She used to knit and do crosswords daily. In the past two years, relatives had begun to notice that she no longer did these activities and that she would often repeat herself in conversations. In the summer her son noticed that she was confused about the use of utensils at lunch. Around the same time Sid hinted several times that May was becoming more confused at home.

In mid-November, Sid was taken ill with a stomach upset, but rather than recovering he stayed in bed for two days and then developed a chest infection that soon became pneumonia. His son and daughter helped to care for him, and without their father helping May, they soon realised that she was very confused and had some form of dementia, possibly Alzheimer's.

Sid's condition got worse rapidly – he had fluid on his heart, had difficulty breathing and his heart was failing. Within a week of falling ill he was admitted into the local Emergency Medical Unit (EMU), but discharged that night when the hospital staff had stabilised him.

At the start of Sid's illness, his daughter contacted the duty social worker at the local social services department and the occupational therapists (OTs) for assistance with aids and adaptations in the house. The social worker visited the couple with their daughter-in-law present and assessed the couple as needing home care three times a day. He explained that for the purposes of the departmental forms and financial assessments, Sid and May's needs had to be assessed separately and potentially two different carers could be visiting them at the same time (as they were viewed as two individual 'service users', not as an interdependent couple). The family knew about the existence of direct payments (cash payments instead of directly provided services) but were told that although this was a possibility, it would take two months to set up. However, changing circumstances meant that the home care was never activated. Sid was admitted back into the EMU later that week and this time he stayed in for several weeks. Meanwhile, his son had contacted May's GP, who was new and had not seen her before. The

GP examined May, suggested a diagnosis of dementia and referred her to a psycho-geriatrician at the local psychiatric unit.

By the time of Sid's second admission, the family had given his details to several different services on several different occasions – to the OTs, to the social workers and to the hospital. The family informed social services that Sid had gone back into hospital. May moved to live with her daughter for the duration of Sid's stay in hospital and spent time with her son and family. She was very disturbed and her son and daughter decided that she could not be left unattended. She was not prone to wandering, but would become agitated when left alone and was losing her sense of danger in household situations. At her daughter's request a social worker from the local office visited May in her daughter's home and thought that she could benefit from some services, mentioning respite care, but did not specify what form this could take.

Once in hospital, Sid's condition did not improve for some weeks; he was very ill with heart failure, but disliked being hospital as it was noisy. He spent two weeks on a ward for patients who had suffered a stroke; one of the other patients was very disturbed and kept most other patients awake at night.

The original social worker from the local office visited Sid in hospital to assess his needs prior to discharge. At this stage he agreed that, if Sid was to return home, both he and May would need 24-hour care, but that this was an ideal solution and that in reality they would get three visits a day from home carers. Just before the Christmas holiday the hospital agreed that Sid could be discharged. The family had not met the social worker face to face, but by phone asked for four or five calls from home carers, including an early morning call to help May get dressed. She was physically able to dress herself, but needed supervision to get washed and to select her clothes. Since Sid's illness, the family realised that he must have been doing this for her for some time. Without an early morning call she would have dressed in any clothes and may have been a danger to herself and others in the kitchen. The social worker could only sanction three calls a day and could not confirm that the first would be before 10am.

However, after a week of negotiating with private agencies the social worker was unable to arrange these calls until 6 January. Sid's son spent much of Christmas Eve talking with the social worker's manager (the worker willingly passed on the responsibility to him when the family complained about the lack of services), ward staff and community staff. He again asked about direct payments and was assured this could be looked at once Sid was home. The OTs and district nurses had carried out assessments and were able to provide services and adaptations. Some of the latter had already been delivered and the family had arranged for a stair lift to be installed in Sid and May's home.

At one stage, Sid's son thought that the NHS Intermediate Care service would be able to provide care until social services were able to take over. Nobody at social services or the hospital ward staff seemed to know about the criteria for this service or how it could be accessed. Eventually, the son found the telephone number of the manager of the service and rang himself. Initially it seemed that this could be the answer, but later that day the manager said that the information given to the son by the GP, ward staff and social services was only partially correct. The Intermediate Care service did exist but only applied to those patients in the community, to prevent their hospital admission, not those awaiting discharge back home. She said that they would be reluctant to offer this service as they had no guarantee that social services would take over once the intermediate care was due to finish. In effect they did not want to take the pressure off social services by facilitating discharges and then be left providing the ongoing care that social services were supposed to provide.

Eventually, late on Christmas Eve, the family agreed to look after Sid until social services could provide two calls a day starting on 2 January (via a private agency). Thereafter the three calls a day would start on 6 January, including a morning call before 9.30am to help May get up, get washed and get dressed. The hospital discharged Sid on Christmas Day and his family and a district nurse were at home to meet him. Sid had developed pressure sores and had a catheter fitted. That night May returned home.

The next day, their children visited them to find that May was becoming more confused and did not always recognise Sid. He had not had much sleep and was in pain. It took his son at least 45 minutes to dress Sid in the morning. From 2 January, one male home carer from a private agency called twice a day at lunchtime and early evening and the pressure on the family eased a little. The family had written a detailed care plan for the carer which he followed well. However, once three calls a day became available, the present carer had to leave as his employers were unable to provide a morning call and the carer was travelling from a neighbouring town (some 10 miles away) to make the lunchtime call. At the best of times, Sid did not like change, and he was reluctant for his present carer to leave as they had built a relationship and were working well together.

Initially, the social worker had reassured Sid's son that the first call would be well before 9.30am once a three-call a day package began. By 3 January, however, he had changed his story and said that there was no way that the first call would be before 9.30am. On 6 January when the new care package was due to start, Sid's daughter-in-law visited at 11.00am to find the couple still in bed as the carer had not turned up. When contacted, the social worker said that carers failing to turn up often happened at the start of a care plan. The social worker himself failed to turn up for an assessment visit later that week, calling in sick in the morning. After pleas for help, the duty social worker came out to do another assessment of Sid and May. He suggested more services that may be appropriate for both, particularly a day centre for May and a visiting service that may take some of the pressure off Sid by providing sitters who would occupy her.

In the following two weeks, Sid and May had 10 different carers from the agency. Towards the end of that period, the agency provided a communication book. No one referred to the care plan the family had produced. Carers did not turn up on another two occasions. Sid's daughter began to spend longer at the house, and as a consequence the carers only spent 15 minutes on each call (two carers for each call as there was lifting to do). At the end of the fortnight a new carer could not cope when Sid collapsed downstairs and dialled 999. Sid was re-admitted to the EMU and transferred to a rehabilitation hospital nearby that weekend.

The social worker told the family that May might be able to stay in the same hospital on a ward for frail relatives. However, after several phone calls to the ward, the family discovered that it could not cope with relatives with Alzheimer's disease. The social worker faxed the son details of nursing homes that could provide respite care for May, but would not make a recommendation about the suitability of any for her. The son contacted those with vacancies and, after a 15-minute visit, arranged for a temporary place at one near to May's house, starting a few days later. The son had still never met the social worker, although his wife and sister had met him once.

Rather than take May into their homes again, the son and daughter had agreed to stay with her in her house should Sid be readmitted to hospital. On the second night of this arrangement, May showed some reluctance to return to her home after spending the day with her son's family. On the third night at about 9.30pm she became aggressive towards her son in his car and then assaulted him. The son did not know what to do. He managed to get his mother into her house, but she was agitated and violent. She was threatening to commit suicide, but also biting and hitting him. He rang her GP and an out-of-hours doctor called at about 11.00pm. He assessed her and decided that she might need to be sectioned under the 1983 Mental Health Act. The assault endured until 2.00am when two approved social workers (ASWs) and a psychiatrist visited and admitted her to the local psychiatric hospital on a Mental Health Act section.

At the time of admission, the staff explained the process to the son and what would happen next. The following day the staff in the unit had arranged meetings with the family, including a counselling session with the unit's psychologist.

Sid's condition deteriorated, and he never left his bed. He died from heart failure in early February. The staff from the psychiatric unit had taken May to see him two days before his death. Shortly after this, May was discharged from the unit to a local nursing home under section 117 of the Mental Health Act (which meant the funding would be the responsibility of the local authority). Despite this, the social services department insisted that the family complete a financial assessment. The reason given by the social worker was that it was so that the department had the information in case May's circumstances changed. The family refused to do this, arguing that it was unnecessary and a waste of time.

May never returned to the place where she had lived since 1947. She had raised her family there, she had been married to Sid since 1940 and their 63rd wedding anniversary was three weeks after his death. The landlord took over the house once the son and daughter had cleared it, gutted it and let it to a family within two months.

Good practice guide

- Assessments and care plans take time, but *do not let bureaucracy take over*. Remember that the focus should be on the needs of the service user and finding out from them and their families what would be most helpful. For many people, this will be their first contact with caring agencies and they will be anxious and frightened about their present situation and the thought of dealing with so many different people and services. Here, workers were working hard, but focusing on administrative procedures and completing forms, some of which were unnecessary. The family had contact with two GPs, two social workers and their manager, two OTs, district nurses, ward staff in several hospitals, psychiatrists, a psychologist, out-of-hours ASWs and a locum doctor. Basic biographical details should not have to be constantly repeated to different workers, especially from the same agency. One person needs to be identified as the coordinator and make links between different agencies.
- Try to take a *holistic view of service users' needs*. Here, the social workers took a very narrow service-focused approach to Sid and May's individual needs. There was little acknowledgement of how Sid and May worked together as a couple and no way of recording this on the assessment forms.
- In your assessments, take a view of possible outcomes and the probability of them happening. Use this as a framework for *contingency planning*. In this case, there was no forward planning or discussion about what would happen if Sid was readmitted to hospital. The family and social workers were always working in a state of crisis and everyone became frustrated and irate.
- Ensure you have *up-to-date information* about what services are available and their eligibility criteria. Be honest with people about what can be provided when, and do not mislead them.
- If you are not appropriately trained, *seek specialist help* with mental health issues. Here, no one seemed to pick up the implications of May's condition and offer appropriate help to the family. The ASWs quickly understood the situation and the pressures on the family and the psychiatric unit offered valuable counselling services immediately.
- Work with *family members as equal partners*. Here the family had done the practical caring and knew what was required, but no one sat down with them and talked about what they could continue to provide and how they could all work together.
- Find out *how service contracts are monitored in your area*. What would be the outcome of services not arriving? Do service users know whom to contact in this event?
- *Do not accept the delivery of mediocre services.* People on the receiving end are relying on you to ensure good quality services which are critical to their quality of life and survival.

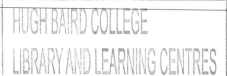

Bibliography and relevant websites

6, P., Leat, D., Seltzer, K. and Stoker, G. (2002) *Towards holistic governance: The new reform agenda*, Basingstoke: Palgrave.

Adams, S. (2001) *On the mend? Hospital discharge services and the role of home improvement agencies*, London: Care and Repair England.

Allen, I., Dalley, G. and Leat, D. (1992) *Monitoring change in social services departments*, London: Policy Studies Institute (for the Association of Directors of Social Services).

Anderson, P., Meara, J., Broadhurst, S., Attwood, S., Timbrell, M. and Gatherer, A. (1988) 'Use of hospital beds: a cohort study of admissions to a provincial teaching hospital', *British Medical Journal*, vol 297, pp 910-12.

Audit Commission (1986) *Making a reality of community care*, London: HMSO.

Audit Commission (1992) *Lying in wait: The use of medical beds in acute hospitals*, London: HMSO.

Audit Commission (1997) *The coming of age: Improving care services for older people*, London: Audit Commission.

Audit Commission (1998) *A fruitful partnership: Effective partnership working*, London: Audit Commission.

Audit Commission (2000) *Forget me not: Mental health services for older people*, London: Audit Commission.

Audit Commission (2002a) *Integrated services for older people: Building a whole systems approach in England*, London: Audit Commission.

Audit Commission (2002b) *Forget me not 2002*, London: Audit Commission.

Balloch, S. and Taylor, M. (eds) (2001) *Partnership working: Policy and practice*, Bristol: The Policy Press.

Banks, P. (2002) *Partnerships under pressure: A commentary on progress in partnership-working between the NHS and local government*, London: King's Fund.

Barnes, D. (1997) *Older people with mental health problems living alone: Anybody's priority?*, London: DoH.

Barnes, M. (1998) 'Frail bodies, courageous voices: older people influencing community care', *Health and Social Care in the Community*, vol 6, no 2, pp 102-11.

Barrett, G. and Hudson, M. (1997) 'Changes in district nursing workload', *Journal of Community Nursing*, vol 11, no 3, pp 4-8.

Bebbington, A. and Charnley, H. (1990) 'Community care for the elderly: rhetoric and reality', *British Journal of Social Work*, vol 20, pp 409-32.

BGS/ADSS/RCN (British Geriatrics Society/Association of Directors of Social Services/Royal College of Nursing)(1995) *The discharge of elderly persons from hospital for community care*, Wolverhampton: BGS/ADSS/RCN.

Bowl, R. (1986) 'Social work with old people', in C. Phillipson and A. Walker (eds) *Ageing and social policy: A critical assessment*, Aldershot: Gower.

Bradley, G. and Manthorpe, J. (eds) (2000) *Working on the fault line*, Birmingham: Venture Press.

Bridges, J., Cotter, A., Meyer, J. and Salvage, A. (2000) 'The progress of older people placed during the first year of the 1996 continuing care guidance', *Health and Social Care in the Community*, vol 8, no 2, pp 147-57.

Brown, L., Tucker, C. and Domokos, T. (2002) *The impact of integrated health and social care teams on older people living in the community*, Bath: University of Bath.

Brown, L., Tucker, C. and Domokos, T. (2003) 'Evaluating the impact of integrated health and social care teams on older people living in the community', *Health and Social Care in the Community*, vol 11, no 2, pp 85-94.

Care Development Group (2001) *Fair care for older people*, Edinburgh: The Stationery Office.

Challis, D. (1999) 'Assessment and care management: developments since the community care reforms', in Royal Commission on Long Term Care *With respect to old age* (Research volume 3), London: The Stationery Office.

Clark, H., Dyer, S. and Horwood, J. (1998) *'That bit of help': the high value of low level preventative services for older people*, Bristol/York: The Policy Press/Joseph Rowntree Foundation.

Clarke, L. (1984) *Domiciliary services for the elderly*, London: Croom Helm.

Clode, D. (2002) 'Another fine mess', *Community Care*, 11-17 June, pp 30-32.

Coid, J. and Crome, P. (1986) 'Bed blocking in Bromley', *British Medical Journal*, vol 292, pp 1253-6.

Coleman, A. and Glendinning, C. (2002) 'Partnerships', in D. Wilkin, A. Coleman, B. Dowling and K. Smith (eds) *National tracker survey of primary care groups and trusts 2001/2002: Taking responsibility?*, Manchester: National Primary Care Research and Development Centre.

Cotter, A., Meyer, J. and Roberts, S. (1998) 'The transition from hospital to long-term institutional care', *Nursing Times*, vol 94, no 34, pp 54-6.

Crawford, A. and Peck, E. (2002) 'Musings, mechanisms and models: exploring partnerships in health and social care', *Mental Health Review*, vol 7, no 2, pp 6-14.

Cumella, S. (1994) *Care management in a primary health care team: An evaluation of the placement of a social worker in the primary health care team at Upton upon Severn*, Birmingham: Birmingham University.

Cumella, S., Le Mesurier, N. and Tomlin, H. (1996) *Social work in practice: An evaluation of the care management received by elderly people from social workers based in GP practices in South Worcestershire*, Martley, Worcestershire: The Martley Press.

DfES/DoH (Department for Education and Skills/Department of Health) (2003) *Together from the start: Practical guidance for professionals working with disabled children (birth to third birthday) and their families*, London: DfES.

Dixon, M., Caulfield, H. and Willis, T. (1999) *Rationing by stealth: A review of the legality of health authorities' continuing care policies in England and Wales*, London: Royal College of Nursing.

DoH (Department of Health) (1989a) *Caring for people: Community care in the next decade and beyond*, London: HMSO.

DoH (1989b) *Working for patients*, London: HMSO.

DoH (1989c) *Discharge of patients from hospital* (guidance booklet accompanying circular HC[89]5, LAC[89]7), London: DoH.

DoH (1990) *Community care in the next decade and beyond: Policy guidance*, London: HMSO.

DoH (1991) *The patient's charter: Raising the standard*, London: HMSO.

DoH (1992a) *Implementing caring for people*, EL(92)13, CI(92)10.

DoH (1992b) *Implementing caring for people*, EL(92)65, CI(92)30.

DoH (1995a) *NHS responsibilities for meeting continuing health care needs*, HSG(95)8, LAC(95)5.

DoH (1995b) *Discharge from NHS inpatient care of people with continuing health or social care needs: Arrangements for reviewing decisions on eligibility for NHS inpatient care*, HSG(95)39, LAC(95)17.

DoH (1995c) *Developing continuing health care policies: A checklist for purchasers*, London: DoH.

DoH (1995d) *Developing and implementing eligibility criteria for continuing health care: A checklist for purchasers*, London: DoH.

DoH (1995e) *NHS responsibilities for meeting continuing health care needs – NHS Executive/SSI monitoring*, EL(95)88, CI(95)37.

DoH (1996a) *NHS responsibilities for meeting continuing health care needs – Current progress and future priorities*, EL(96)8, CI(96)5.

DoH (1996b) *Progress in practice: Initial evaluation of the impact of the continuing care guidance*, EL(96)89, CI(96)35.

DoH (1996c) *Funding for priority services 1996/97 and 1997/98*, EL(96)109.

DoH (1997a) *Managing winter 1997/98*, MISC(97)62.

DoH (1997b) *NHS finance – Additional money for patient care*, EL(97)61.

DoH (1997c) *Better services for vulnerable people*, EL(97)62, CI(97)24.

DoH (1997d) *Community care – Special Transitional Grant conditions and indicative allocations 1998/99*, LASSL(97)25.

DoH (1997e) *The new NHS: Modern, dependable*, London: The Stationery Office.

DoH (1997f) *Our healthier nation: A contract for health*, London: The Stationery Office.

DoH (1998a) *Partnership in action: New opportunities for joint working between health and social services – A discussion document*, London: DoH.

DoH (1998b) *Modernising social services: Promoting independence, improving protection, raising standards*, London: The Stationery Office.

DoH (1999a) *Saving lives: Our healthier nation*, London: The Stationery Office.

DoH (1999b) *Statement on Coughlan judgement*, DoH press release, 16 July.

DoH (1999c) *Ex parte Coughlan: Follow up action*, HSC 1999/180, LAC(99)30.

DoH (2000a) *Winter 2000/01: Capacity planning for health and social care*, HSC 2000/016, LAC(2000)14.

DoH (2000b) *The NHS plan: The government's response to the Royal Commission on Long Term Care*, London: The Stationery Office.

DoH (2000c) *The NHS plan: A plan for investment, a plan for reform*, London: The Stationery Office.

DoH (2001a) *2001/2002: Arrangements for whole system capacity planning – Emergency, elective and social care*, HSC 2001/014, LAC(2001)17.

DoH (2001b) *Continuing care: NHS and local councils' responsibilities*, HSC 2001/015, LAC(2001)18.

DoH (2001c) *Guide to integrating community equipment stores*, London: DoH.

DoH (2001d) *Community equipment services*, HSC 2001/008, LAC(2001)13.

DoH (2001e) *Intermediate care*, HSC 2001/001, LAC (2001)1.

DoH (2001f) *National service framework for older people: Modern standards and service models*, London: DoH.

DoH (2001g) *Guidance on free NHS funded nursing care in nursing homes*, HSC 2001/17, LAC(2001)26.

DoH (2001h) *The single assessment process: Consultation papers and progress* (www.doh.gov.uk/scg/sap/, accessed 20/08/2001).

DoH (2001i) *Care trusts: Emerging framework*, London: DoH.

DoH (2001j) *Shifting the balance of power within the NHS: Securing delivery*, London: DoH.

DoH (2001k) *£300 million 'cash for change' initiative to tackle 'bedblocking'*, Press Release 2001/0464, London: DoH.

DoH (2001l) *Building capacity and partnership in care: An agreement between the statutory and the independent social care, health care and housing sectors*, London: DoH.

DoH (2002a) *Learning disabilities: Good practice guidance on partnership working* (www.doh.gov.uk/learningdisabilities/partnership/, accessed 31/10/2002).

DoH (2002b) *Delivering the NHS plan: Next steps on investment, next steps on reform*, London: DoH.

DoH (2002c) *Intermediate care: Moving forward*, London: DoH.

DoH (2003a) *Guidance on NHS funded nursing care*, HSC 2003/006, LAC(2003)7.

DoH (2003b) *Guidance on access and systems capacity grant 2003/04*, LAC(2003)10.

DoH (2003c) *Change agent team* (www.doh.gov.uk/changeagentteam/, accessed 25/04/2003).

DoH (2003d) *Discharge from hospital: Pathway, process and practice*, London: DoH.

DoH (2003e) *The Community Care (Delayed Discharges etc) Act 2003: Guidance for implementation*, London: DoH.

DoH/SSI (Department of Health/Social Services Inspectorate) (1991a) *Care management and assessment: Practitioners' guide*, London: HMSO.

DoH/SSI (1991b) *Care management and assessment: Managers' guide*, London: HMSO.

DoH/SSI (1991c) *Care management and assessment: Summary of practice guidance*, London: HMSO.

DoH/SSI (1992) *Social services for hospital patients I: Working at the interface*, London: DoH.

DoH/SSI (1995a) *Moving on: Report of the national inspection of social services department arrangements for the discharge of older people from hospital to residential or nursing home care*, London: DoH.

DoH/SSI (1995b) *Caring for people at home: An overview of the national inspection of social services department arrangements for the assessment and delivery of home care services*, London: DoH.

DoH/SSI (1996) *Caring for people at home – Part II: Report of a second inspection of arrangements for assessment and delivery of home care services*, London: DoH.

DoH/SSI (1997) *At home with dementia: Inspection of services for older people with dementia in the community*, London: DoH.

Dominelli, L. (1988) *Anti-racist social work*, Basingstoke: Macmillan.

Dyer, C. (1998) 'Judge rules NHS cannot jettison long-term care', *The Guardian*, 12 December.

Foote, C. and Stanners, C. (2002) *Integrating care for older people: New care for old – A systems approach*, London: Jessica Kingsley.

George, M. (1996) 'Pass the patient', *Community Care*, 14 March, pp 20-1.

Glasby, J. (2002a) 'Charging ahead', *Nursing Older People*, vol 13, no 1, p 7.

Glasby, J. (2002b) 'The wrong remedy', *Community Care*, 5-11 December, pp 36-7.

Glasby, J. (ed) (2002c) *Acute concerns: Responding to delayed discharges and 'blocked beds'*, Birmingham: Health Services Management Centre.

Glasby, J. (2003a) *Hospital discharge: Integrating health and social care*, Oxon: Radcliffe Medical Press.

Glasby, J. (2003b) 'Planning and preparing for intermediate care', in S. Wade (ed) *Intermediate care and older people*, London: Whurr Publications.

Glasby, J. (2003c) 'Delayed reaction', *Community Care*, 10-16 July, pp 38-9.

Glasby, J. and Littlechild, R. (2002) *Social work and direct payments*, Bristol: The Policy Press.

Glasby, J. and Peck, E. (eds) (2003) *Care trusts: Partnership working in action*, Oxon: Radcliffe Medical Press.

Glasby, J., Littlechild, R. and Pryce, K. (2003) *Show me the way to go home: Delayed hospital discharges and older people*, Birmingham: Health Services Management Centre/Institute of Applied Social Studies.

Glendinning, C. (2002) 'A charge too far', *Community Care*, 11-17 July, pp 34-6.

Glendinning, C., Powell, M. and Rummery, K. (2002a) *Partnerships, New Labour and the governance of welfare*, Bristol: The Policy Press.

Glendinning, C., Hudson, B., Hardy, B. and Young, R. (2002b) *National evaluation of notifications for the use of the Section 31 partnership flexibilities in the Health Act 1999: Final project report*, Leeds/Manchester: Nuffield Institute for Health/National Primary Care Research and Development Centre.

Godfrey, M., Randall, T., Long, A. and Grant, M. (2000) *Review of effectiveness and outcomes: Home care*, Exeter: Centre for Evidence-Based Practice.

Godlove, C. and Mann, A. (1980) 'Thirty years of the welfare state: current issues in British social policy for the aged', *Aged Care and Services Review*, vol 2, no 1, pp 1-12.

Goodwin, N. and Shapiro, J. (2001) *The road to integrated care working* (Research Report no 39), Birmingham: Health Services Management Centre.

Griffiths, R. (1988) *Community care: Agenda for action. A report to the Secretary of State for Social Services by Sir Roy Griffiths*, London: HMSO.

Hancock, M., Villeneau, L. and Hill, R. (1997) *Together we stand: Effective partnerships – Key indicators for joint working in mental health*, London: Sainsbury Centre for Mental Health.

Hardy, B., Hudson, B. and Waddington, E. (2000) *What makes a good partnership? A partnership assessment tool*, Leeds: Nuffield Institute for Health/NHS Executive Trent Region.

Health Service Ombudsman (2003) *NHS funding for long term care*, London: The Stationery Office.

Henwood, M. (1990) *Community care and older people: Policy, practice and research review*, London: Family Policy Studies Centre.

Henwood, M. (1992) 'Twilight zone', *Health Service Journal*, 5 November, pp 28-30.

Henwood, M. (ed) (1994) *Hospital discharge workbook: A manual on hospital discharge practice*, London: DoH.

Henwood, M. (1995) 'Strained relations', *Health Service Journal*, 6 July, pp 22-3.

Henwood, M. (2000) 'Central–local relations: the changing balance', in B. Hudson (ed) *The changing role of social care*, London: Jessica Kingsley.

Henwood, M. and Waddington, E. (2000) *Messages and findings from the Outcomes of Social Care for Adults (OSCA) programme*, Leeds: Nuffield Institute for Health.

Henwood, M. and Wistow, G. (1993) *Hospital discharge and community care: Early days*, Leeds: Nuffield Institute for Health.

Henwood, M., Lewis, H. and Waddington, E. (1998) *Listening to users of domiciliary care services*, Leeds: Nuffield Institute for Health.

Henwood, M., Hardy, B., Hudson, B. and Wistow, G. (1997) *Interagency collaboration: Hospital discharge and continuing care sub-study*, Leeds: Nuffield Institute for Health.

Hill, M. and Macgregor, G. (2001) *Health's forgotten partners? How carers are supported through hospital discharge*, London: Carers UK.

Hiscock, J. and Pearson, M. (1999) 'Looking inwards, looking outwards: dismantling the "Berlin Wall" between health and social services?', *Social Policy and Administration*, vol 33, no 2, pp 150-63.

HM Treasury (2003) *Every child matters*, London: The Stationery Office.

Holtom, M. (2001) 'The partnership imperative: joint working between social services and health', *Journal of Management in Medicine*, vol 15, no 6, pp 430-45.

Holzhausen, E. (2001) *'You can take him home now': Carers' experiences of hospital discharge*, London: Carers National Association.

Horne, D. (1998) *Getting better? Inspection of hospital discharge (care management) arrangements for older people*, London: DoH.

House of Commons Debates (1997) *Hansard*, 9 December, col 802.

House of Commons Health Committee (1999) *The relationship between health and social services*, First Report, London: The Stationery Office.

House of Commons Health Committee (2002) *Delayed discharges*, London: The Stationery Office.

House of Commons Social Services Committee (1985) *Second report: Community care*, House of Commons Paper 13-1, Session 1984-85, London: HMSO.

Hudson, B. (2000) 'Interagency collaboration: a sceptical view', in A. Brechin, H. Brown and M.A. Eby (eds) *Critical practice in health and social care*, Milton Keynes: Open University Press.

Hudson, B. and Henwood, M. (2002) 'The NHS and social care: the final countdown?', *Policy & Politics*, vol 30, no 2, pp 153-66.

Hudson, B., Hardy, B., Henwood, M. and Wistow, G. (1997) *Interagency collaboration: Final report*, Leeds: Nuffield Institute for Health.

Hunter, M. (1999) 'Pressure mounts on government to clarify arrangements for long-term nursing care', *Community Care*, 22-28 July, pp 4-5.

Huws Jones, R. (1952) 'Old people's welfare – successes and failures', *Social Service Quarterly*, vol 26, no 1, pp 19-22.

King's Fund (2002) *Rehabilitation and intermediate care publications* (www.kingsfund.org.uk/eHealthSocialCare/html/rehab_publications.html, accessed 24/04/2003).

Koffman, J., Fulop, N., Pashley, D. and Coleman, K. (1996) 'No way out: the delayed discharge of elderly mentally ill acute and assessment patients in North and South Thames regions', *Age and Ageing*, vol 25, no 4, pp 268-72.

Lacey, P. (2001) *Support partnerships: Collaboration in action*, London: David Fulton Publishers.

Laming, H. (2003) *The Victoria Climbie Inquiry*, London: HMSO.

Le Mesurier, N. and Cumella, S. (1996) *Social work at Tile Hill primary health care services: An evaluation of a social worker secondment to five practices in West Coventry*, Birmingham: Birmingham University.

Le Mesurier, N. and Cumella, S. (2001) 'The rough road and the smooth road: comparing access to social care for older people via area teams and GP surgeries', *Managing Community Care*, vol 9, no 1, pp 7-13.

Leathard, A. (ed) (1994) *Going inter-professional: Working together for health and welfare*, London: Routledge.

Leathard, A. (ed) (2003) *Inter-professional collaboration: From policy to practice in health and social care*, London: Brunner-Routledge.

Leutz, W. (1999) 'Five laws for integrating medical and social services: lessons from the US and UK', *Milbank Quarterly*, vol 77, no 1, pp 77-110.

Lewis, J. (2001) 'Older people and the health–social care boundary in the UK: half a century of hidden policy conflict', *Social Policy and Administration*, vol 35, no 4, pp 343-59.

Littlechild, R., Smallwood, H., Jeffes, L. and Chesterman, M. (1995) 'Care management for older people discharged from hospital', *Elders*, vol 4, no 4, pp 37-50.

Local Government Association (2000) *Partnerships with health: A survey of local authorities*, London: Local Government Association.

Lowndes, V. and Skelcher, C. (1998) 'The dynamics of multi-organizational partnerships: an analysis of changing modes of governance', *Public Administration*, vol 76, pp 313-33.

Loxley, A. (1997) *Collaboration in health and welfare*, London: Jessica Kingsley.

Malin, V. (2000) 'From continuous to continuing long-term care', in G. Bradley and J. Manthorpe (eds) *Working on the fault line*, Birmingham: Venture Press.

Marks, L. (1994) *Seamless care or patchwork quilt? Discharging patients from acute hospital care*, Research Report 17, London: King's Fund Institute.

Marshall, M. (1990) 'Proud to be old', in E. McEwen (ed) *Age: The unrecognised discrimination*, London: Age Concern England.

Meads, G. (ed) (1997) *Health and social services in primary care: An effective combination?*, London: Financial Times Healthcare.

Means, R. (1986) 'The development of social services: historical perspectives', in C. Phillipson and A. Walker (eds) *Ageing and social policy: A critical assessment*, Aldershot: Gower.

Means, R. and Smith, R. (1998a) *Community care: Policy and practice* (2nd edn), Basingstoke: Macmillan.

Means, R. and Smith, R. (1998b) *From poor law to community care: The development of welfare services for elderly people, 1939-1971* (2nd edn), Bristol: The Policy Press.

Means, R., Morbey, H. and Smith, R. (2002) *From community care to market care? The development of welfare services for older people*, Bristol: The Policy Press.

Means, R., Richards, S. and Smith, R. (2003) *Community care: Policy and practice* (3rd edn), Basingstoke: Palgrave Macmillan.

MoH (Ministry of Health) (1957a) *Local authority services for the chronic sick and infirm*, 14/57.

MoH (1957b) *Geriatric services and the care of the chronic sick*, HM(57)86.

Murphy, E. (1977) 'Blocked beds', *British Medical Journal*, vol i, pp 1395-6.

National Audit Office (2000) *Inpatient admissions and bed management in NHS acute hospitals*, London: The Stationery Office.

NAO (National Audit Office) (2003) *Ensuring the effective discharge of older patients from NHS acute hospitals*, London: The Stationery Office.

Neill, J. and Williams, J. (1992) *Leaving hospital: Older people and their discharge to community care*, London: HMSO.

NHSE (National Health Service Executive) (1998) *Unlocking the potential: Effective partnerships for improving health*, London: NHSE.

Nocon, A. (1994) *Collaboration in community care in the 1990s*, Sunderland: Business Education Publishers.

Nocon, A. and Baldwin, S. (1998) *Trends in rehabilitation policy: A review of the literature*, London: King's Fund.

Norman, I.J. and Peck, E. (1999) 'Working together in adult community mental health services: an inter-professional dialogue', *Journal of Mental Health*, vol 8, no 3, pp 217-30.

O'Hagan, G. (1999) *Of primary importance: Inspection of social services departments' links with primary health services – Older people*, London: DoH.

Øvretveit, J., Mathias, P. and Thompson, T. (eds) (1997) *Interprofessional working for health and social care*, Basingstoke: Macmillan.

Pattie, A. and Heaton, J. (1990) *A comparative study of dependency and provision of care for the elderly in the state and private sectors in York health district*, York: Yorkshire Regional Health Authority.

Payne, M. (2000) *Teamwork in multiprofessional care*, Basingstoke: Macmillan.

Peck, E. and Norman, I.J. (1999) 'Working together in adult community mental health services: exploring inter-professional role relations', *Journal of Mental Health*, vol 8, no 3, pp 231-42.

Peck, E., Gulliver, P. and Towell, D. (2002a) *Modernising partnerships: An evaluation of Somerset's innovations in the commissioning and organisation of mental health services – Final report*, London: Institute of Applied Health and Social Policy, King's College.

Peck, E., Gulliver, P. and Towell, D. (2002b) 'Governance of partnership between health and social services: the experience in Somerset', *Health and Social Care in the Community*, vol 10, no 5, pp 331-9.

Peck, E., Towell, D. and Gulliver, P. (2001) 'The meanings of "culture" in health and social care: a case study of the combined trust in Somerset', *Journal of Interprofessional Care*, vol 15, no 4, pp 319-27.

Petch, A. (2003) *Intermediate care: What do we know about older people's experiences?*, York: Joseph Rowntree Foundation.

Phillipson, J. and Williams, J. (1995) *Action on hospital discharge*, London: National Institute of Social Work.

Poxton, R. (1999) *Partnerships in primary and social care: Integrating services for vulnerable people*, London: King's Fund.

Poxton, R. (2003) 'What makes effective partnerships between health and social care?', in J. Glasby and E. Peck (eds) *Care trusts: Partnership working in action*, Oxon: Radcliffe Medical Press.

Pratt, J., Plampling, D. and Gordon, P. (1998) *Partnership: Fit for purpose?*, Whole Systems Thinking Working Paper Series, London: King's Fund.

Quilgars, D. (2000) *Low intensity support services*, Bristol: The Policy Press.

RADAR (2003) *Crossing the boundaries: How training can improve joint working*, London: RADAR.

Raynes, N., Temple, B., Glenister, C. and Coulthard, L. (2001) *Quality at home for older people*, Bristol/York: The Policy Press/Joseph Rowntree Foundation.

Roberts, P. and Houghton, M. (1996) 'In search of a block buster', *Health Service Journal*, 5 December, pp 28-9.

Royal Commission on Long Term Care (1999) *With respect to old age: Long term care – Rights and responsibilities*, London: The Stationery Office.

Royal Commission on Long Term Care (2003) *Long-term care: Statement by Royal Commissioners*, London: The Stationery Office.

Rubin, S. and Davies, G. (1975) 'Bed blocking by elderly patients in general hospital wards', *Age and Ageing*, vol 4, pp 142-7.

Rummery, K. and Glendinning, C. (2000) *Primary care and social services: Developing new partnerships for older people*, Oxon: Radcliffe Medical Press.

Sainsbury Centre for Mental Health (2000) *Taking your partners: Using opportunities for interagency partnership in mental health*, London: Sainsbury Centre for Mental Health.

Shaw, T. (1998) 'Paralysed resident of home wins care case', *The Daily Telegraph*, 12 December.

Sidell, M. (1995) *Health in old age: Myth, mystery and management*, Buckingham: Open University Press.

Sinclair, A. and Dickinson, E. (1998) *Effective practice in rehabilitation: Evidence from systematic reviews*, London: King's Fund.

Sinclair, I. and Williams, J. (1990) 'Domiciliary services', in I. Sinclair, R. Parker, D. Leat and J. Williams (eds) *The kaleidoscope of care: A review of research on welfare provision for elderly people*, London: HMSO.

Sinclair, I., Gibbs, I. and Hicks, L. (2000) *The management and effectiveness of the home care service*, York: The University of York.

Sinclair, I., Parker, R., Leat, D. and Williams, J. (1990) *The kaleidoscope of care: A review of research on welfare provision for elderly people*, London: HMSO.

Smallwood, H. and Jeffes, L. (nd) *Hereford hospital discharge project*, Unpublished Report, Hereford and Worcester County Council Social Services Department.

Smith, H., Pryce, A., Carlisle, L., Jones, J., Scarpello, J. and Pantin, C. (1997) 'Appropriateness of acute medical admissions and length of stay', *Journal of the Royal College of Physicians of London*, vol 31, no 5, pp 527-32.

South, J. (1999) 'Eligibility criteria and entitlements: defining need for NHS continuing care', *Social Policy and Administration*, vol 33, no 2, pp 132-49.

Sullivan, H. and Skelcher, C. (2002) *Working across boundaries: Collaboration in public services*, Basingstoke: Palgrave.

Tanner, D. (2001) 'Partnership in prevention: messages from older people', in V. White and J. Harris (eds) *Developing good practice in community care*, London: Jessica Kingsley Publishers.

Thompson, N. (2001) *Anti-discriminatory practice* (3rd edn), Basingstoke: Palgrave.

Tinker, A. (1997) *Older people in modern society* (4th edn), London: Longman.

Towell, D. (2002) *Partnership Boards and user engagement: What do you think of the show so far?*, London: Foundation for People with Learning Disabilities (www.learningdisabilities.org.uk/html/content/pftopic09.cfm, accessed 29/11/2002).

Tucker, C. and Brown, L. (1997) *Moving towards integration: An evaluation of different models for accessing community care services for adults and their carers*, Bath: University of Bath.

Twigg, J. (1997) 'Deconstructing the "social bath": help with bathing at home for older and disabled people', *Journal of Social Policy*, vol 26, no 2, pp 211-32.

Vaughan, B. and Lathlean, B. (1999) *Intermediate care: Models in practice*, London: King's Fund.

Victor, C. (1997) *Community care and older people*, Cheltenham: Stanley Thornes.

Walters, B. (2001) 'Working with health: partnership in a community setting', in V. White and J. Harris (eds) *Developing good practice in community care*, London: Jessica Kingsley Publishers.

Warren, M. (1951) 'The elderly in the community', *Social Service Quarterly*, vol 24, no 3, pp 102-6.

Watson, D., Townsley, R., Abbott, D. and Latham, P. (2002) *Working together? Multi-agency working in services to disabled children with complex health needs and their families: A literature review*, Birmingham: Handsel Trust.

Wilkin, D., Coleman, A., Dowling, B. and Smith, K. (eds) (2002) *National tracker survey of primary care groups and trusts 2001/2002: Taking responsibility?*, Manchester: National Primary Care Research and Development Centre.

Wistow, G. (1996) The changing scene in Britain', in T. Harding, B. Meredith and G. Wistow (eds) *Options for long term care: Economic, social and ethical choices*, London: HMSO.

Wistow, G. and Fuller, S. (1982) *Joint planning in perspective*, Birmingham: Centre for Research in Social Policy and National Association of Health Authorities.

Wistow, G., Hardy, B., Henwood, M. and Hudson, B. (1997) 'Interagency collaboration: links between primary health care and social services', *Update*, no 3, Leeds: Nuffield Institute for Health.

Relevant websites

Age Concern	www.ace.org.uk
Association of Directors of Social Services	www.adss.org.uk
Audit Commission	www.auditcommission.gov.uk
Community Care	www.communitycare.co.uk
Department of Health	www.dh.gov.uk
Health Service Journal	www.hsj.co.uk
Health Services Management Centre	www.bham.ac.uk/hsmc
Help the Aged	www.helptheaged.org.uk
House of Commons Health Committee	www.parliament.uk/commons/ selcom/hlthhome.htm
Integrated Care Network	www.integratedcarenetwork.gov.uk
King's Fund	www.kingsfund.org.uk
Local Government Association	www.lga.gov.uk
NHS Confederation	www.nhsconfed.org/
National Evaluation of Intermediate Care	www.prw.le.ac.uk/intcare
Nuffield Institute for Health	www.nuffield.leeds.ac.uk
Nursing Older People	www.nursing-standard.co.uk/ olderpeople

Index

Page references for notes are followed by n